D1214232

COLOR ATLAS OF GROSS PLACENTAL PATHOLOGY

COLOR ATLAS OF GROSS PLACENTAL PATHOLOGY

Cynthia G. Kaplan, M.D.
Associate Professor of Pathology
Department of Pathology
State University of New York at Stony Brook
Stony Brook, New York

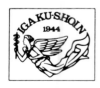

IGAKU-SHOIN   New York • Tokyo

Published and distributed by

IGAKU-SHOIN Medical Publishers, Inc.
One Madison Avenue, New York, New York 10010

IGAKU-SHOIN Ltd.,
5-24-3 Hongo, Bunkyo-ku, Tokyo 113-91.

Library of Congress Cataloging-in-Publication Data

Kaplan, Cynthia G.
    Color atlas of gross placental pathology / Cynthia G. Kaplan.
      p. cm.
    Includes bibliographical references and index.
    ISBN 0-89640-249-5
    1. Placenta—Diseases—Atlases. 2. Placenta—Abnormalities—
Atlases. I. Title.
    [DNLM: 1. Placenta—pathology—atlases. WQ 17 K17c 1994]
  RG591.K37   1994
  618.3′4—dc20
  DNLM/DLC
  for Library of Congress   93-33096
                                               CIP

ISBN: 0-89640-249-5 (New York)
ISBN: 4-260-14249-6 (Tokyo)

Printed and bound in the U.S.A.

10 9 8 7 6 5 4 3 2 1

DEDICATION

To my family, without whose support this would not have been possible, to Kurt Benirschke who started me on this path, and to the memory of Lauren Ackerman, who had been a great supporter of my work.

ACKNOWLEDGMENTS

I would like to acknowledge the assistance of those individuals in the pathology laboratory who have helped me over the years with my examinations of placentas, and encouraged me to write this book. Media Services at State University of New York, Stony Brook ably processed all the illustrative material.

PREFACE

Careful evaluation of the placenta can often give much insight into disorders of pregnancy in the mother and fetus. It can confirm the clinical suspicion of processes such as hemorrhage or infection, explain problems during labor, and lead to specific diagnoses in cases of hydrops, growth retardation, or fetal demise. The placenta also holds clues to the origins of disease unsuspected at birth, manifesting later with significant sequelae.

Frequently the placenta has been examined only cursorily and then discarded. This is unfortunate. Many clinically significant macroscopic lesions can be readily identified with a minimum of effort. Additionally, the gross examination often suggests the presence of microscopic abnormalities. Fortunately change is occurring in the handling of placentas. Thorough gross evaluation of placentas from all deliveries is now promoted, with triage for histology of those from pregnancies with significant clinical history or with abnormal initial examination.

The techniques of gross placental examination are not difficult, but a systematic approach is necessary to be complete. While it is possible for others to review microscopic slides, the gross findings will exist only as originally observed and recorded. This book is designed to aid in careful and thorough gross examination by providing the images and vocabulary required. It depicts normal variations and common abnormal findings, with some examples of more unusual pathology as well. Fresh specimens are used predominantly, as placentas are always examined in this state in the delivery room, and frequently in pathology as well. Lesions are presented by site rather than by diseases process, since this is how one actually encounters them in the course of doing the placental evaluation. Important clinicopathologic correlations and related histopathology for major processes are included. Normal tables, selected references, and sample forms are found in the appendices.

This material is drawn from the examination of over 20,000 placentas delivered since the opening of University Hospital, Stony Brook in 1980. Gross photography was done in the surgical pathology suite using a copystand and a 35mm camera with a Nikon 55mm 1:1 macro lens. Ektachrome 64 and 100 daylight film were used, with processing done on the premises.

Cynthia G. Kaplan, M.D.

CONTENTS

1
EXAMINATION PROCEDURES

SITE

The two most likely locations for the initial gross placental examination are the delivery room and the pathology suite. This exam need not be done by a pathologist or obstetrician. It can be performed by other trained personnel such as nurses, or physician's assistants. Based on the history and the initial evaluation, the responsible individual sends all abnormal or potentially abnormal placentas for full gross and microscopic examination. Although the initial triage exam may not be as complete as the gross examination outlined below, it should be reasonably thorough and include measurements of cord and placental size, as well as careful observation and palpation.

INDICATIONS FOR HISTOLOGY

There are maternal, fetal, and placental indications for histology (Table 1-1). The number of placentas examined microscopically will vary with the nature of the obstetrical population, but is unlikely to be less than 5–10%. It has been argued that all placentas should be examined microscopically because a significant percentage of children with later problems cannot be predicted from obstetrical and neonatal history. An intermediate solution is to archive tissue or blocks. For example, those placentas not initially selected for microscopic examination still have the standard (three) blocks processed. These are stored permanently and can be cut if indicated.

FIXATION

The question of whether to examine placentas fresh or fixed has long been debated, without a definite answer. The fresh placenta permits microbiologi-

Table 1-1.   Indications for Placental Histology

Fetal/Neonatal	Maternal
Stillbirth/perinatal death	Maternal disorders (e.g. hypertension, collagen disease, diabetes, drug abuse)
Hydrops	
Multiple gestation	
Prematurity (<35 weeks)	Possible infection/fever
Postmaturity (>42 weeks)	Poor reproductive history
Intrauterine growth retardation	Abruptio placenta
Congenital anomalies (major)	Repetitive bleeding
Possible infection	Oligohydramnios
Seizures	Polyhydramnios
Admission to Neonatal Intensive Care Unit (NICU)	
Compromised condition at birth (e.g. low pH or Apgar scores)	

Placental
Abnormal fetal/placental weight
  ratio
Extensive infarction
Single umbilical artery
Meconium staining
Suggestive of infection
Retroplacental hemorrhage
Excessive fibrin deposition
Villous atrophy
Chorangioma
Amnion nodosum

cal cultures, frozen section, and the establishment of cell culture for karyotype or other testing. Surface changes are better appreciated and membrane rolls are easily made. It is also more readily palpated for solid lesions. Injection studies in twins can only be done on fresh placentas. Unfixed placentas may be held for several days refrigerated prior to gross examination. Gross and microscopic changes are minimal, if any, over this time. The fixed placenta is more simply transported and stored, is less infectious, and may show infarcted regions better. Good fixation of an intact placenta will require several days' immersion in several times its volume of formalin.

TECHNIQUE OF GROSS EXAMINATION

Complete gross examinations of placentas can be done quite rapidly with some experience. Placentas, whether fresh or fixed, are large, messy specimens and more comfortably handled in an easily cleaned area, such as a table with running water. If the placenta is initially examined fresh, represen-

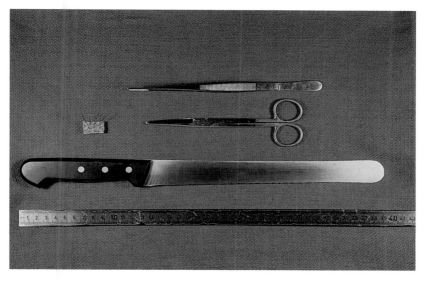

Figure 1-1. Implements useful for gross placental examination include a large thin round-ended knife for the major cutting, a metal meter stick for measurements, a long thin forceps with delicate teeth for membranes rolls, pins to hold the rolls intact in formalin, and a scissors for trimming. A hanging pan balance is most convenient for weighing.

tative portions should be fixed for at least a day prior to the final blocking. The remainder of the placenta can be discarded, except for those placentas with very unusual findings.

Gross examination of placentas should be done in a fixed routine, so all features are assessed. Certain easily obtainable instruments simplify the process (Figure 1-1). It is also useful to have an assistant who notes data on a specialized form (Appendix A-1). The following briefly summarizes the steps. Specific findings are detailed in subsequent chapters.

1. The placental exam begins on opening the container. In fresh placentas an unusual odor may indicate bacterial infection. Large amounts of fresh clot suggest the possibility of premature separation (abruption).
2. The general shape of the placenta is assessed and extra lobes noted. The fetal surface is examined for color, fibrin deposition, subchorionic and subamniotic hemorrhages, cysts, vascular pattern, and blood vessel changes such as thrombi (Figure 1-2). The maternal surface is inspected for color, completeness, and adherent blood clot. The villous tissue is palpated for lesions (Figure 1-3).
3. The cord is measured and its site of insertion in the placental disk noted. Particular attention should be given to the presence and intactness of velamentous vessels.
4. The cord is inspected for true knots, twisting, and discolorations. It is then cut several centimeters from its placental insertion and the cut

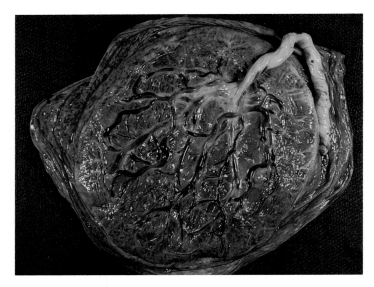

Figure 1-2. Intact fresh normal term placenta showing the fetal surface. The cord is present inserting just off center. The surface is bluish with no opacification or unusual coloration. Subchorionic fibrin, usual in mature placentas, leads to the whiter areas. Free peripheral membranes can be seen at the margin.

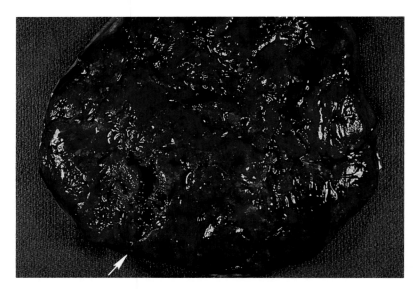

Figure 1-3. The maternal surface of a term placenta shows intact villous tissue except for a small area of disruption (*arrow*), which could indicate tissue has been left in the uterus. The placental cotyledons are vaguely outlined. A small amount of loose, soft, postpartum clot is present (2 and 5 o'clock) which should be removed prior to weighing and further examination. There are small white flecks of calcium.

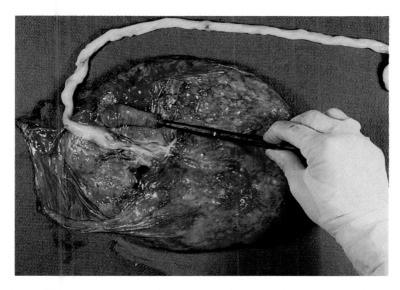

Figure 1-4. The membranes of this normal, term placenta have been placed in their *in situ* uterine position. With a vaginal delivery, the minimal distance from the hole of rupture to the edge of the placental disk indicates the site of the placenta in the uterus. Shorter lengths indicate low-lying placentas. The membrane roll is made from the rupture point to the margin of the placenta. It is then pinned, cut, and fixed.

    end examined for the number of vessels and other abnormalities. Portions of the cord from the proximal and distal regions are fixed.

5. The peripheral membranes are inverted if necessary, and lifted into their anatomic position with maternal surface exterior. They are inspected for the type of insertion into the disk, completeness, and the distance of the point of rupture from the edge of the placenta. The color, opacity, and other lesions such as hemorrhages and compressed twins are noted.

6. A strip of membranes (about 4 cm wide) is cut from the edge of the site of rupture to the margin of the disk. A "jellyroll" is made by grasping the end with long thin forceps and rolling toward the placenta. This puts the point of rupture at the center of the roll, which is held in place with a pin and cut from the placenta. The pin is unnecessary with hardening fixatives such as Bouin's. Rolls are difficult to make once the placenta has been fixed or if the membranes are severely disrupted or "slimy" from meconium (Figures 1-4 and 1-5).

7. The remaining membranes are trimmed away (with scissors or knife) and any loose soft clot is removed from the maternal surface. The placenta is now weighed, without cord or membranes, in a hanging pan balance. Measurements are taken of greatest diameters and thickness, and any extra lobes.

8. Transverse cuts are made through the maternal surface at 1- to 2-cm

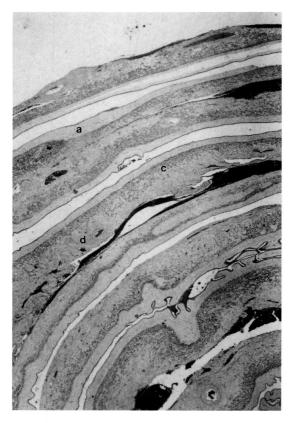

Figure 1-5. Histologic section of a cross section of a membrane roll shows the numerous layers visible by this technique. Amnion (a), chorion (c), and attached decidua (d) with small blood vessels are present.

       intervals. Lesions are measured and described. The degree of calcification and any unusual features such as villous color or texture are noted (Figure 1-6).
  9. Representative pieces of the placenta are cut and fixed, to include margin, central villi from several cotyledons, and any significant gross lesions (Figure 1-7).

PLACENTAL WEIGHT

Placental weight varies with the methodology of weighing. It is affected by fixation, the presence of cord, membranes, and loose clot, the amount of blood retained, and the intactness of the maternal surface. Fresh refrigerated placentas lose a small amount of weight with storage, whereas formalin fixation leads to an increase. The value of placental weight is largely at the

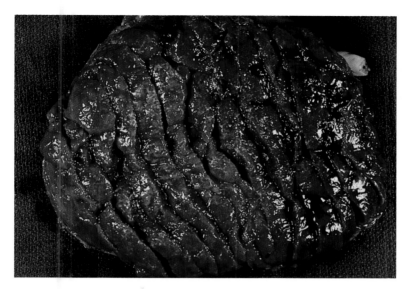

Figure 1-6. Mature placenta after 1–1.5 cm transverse cuts have been made on the maternal surface in order to examine the villous tissue. The fetal surface is not usually cut and keeps the placenta intact.

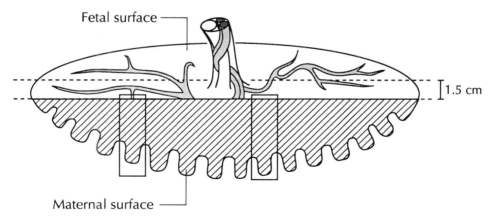

Figure 1-7. The placental villous tissue routinely fixed and saved is a transverse strip from the central region, which will often include the cord. This piece should be about 1.5 cm wide for adequate fixation. Histologic blocks of villous tissue are taken from two separate areas in the placental midzone, as indicated by the boxes. Tissue near the margin shows substantial artifact due to poor perfusion in this region. Blocks ideally include small surface vessels and do not have thick subchorionic fibrin.

extremes, taking into account the gestational age and weight of the baby. A relatively heavy or light placenta often indicates an abnormal pregnancy. At term, the infant usually weighs about 7–8 times the placental weight. The ratio decreases earlier in gestation. Most term placentas weighing more than 750 grams or less than 350 grams warrant histology. There are standard tables for weight and fetal–placental ratio (Appendices B-1, B-2, and B-3).

HISTOLOGIC SECTIONING

Although it is possible to block a fresh placenta, this is far easier after overnight fixation. Sharp blades are important to keep the amnion on the placental surface intact. On most placentas three blocks with cord, membrane roll, and two full thickness pieces of villous tissue including fetal and maternal surfaces are adequate. The two pieces of placental tissue should be from separate areas (different cotyledons), and *not* from the margin of the placenta, which frequently shows changes of diminished blood flow (Figure 1-7). The fetal surface of the section should include small blood vessels, and be free of substantial subchorionic clot or fibrin. Early changes of ascending infection are often masked in areas with thick subchorionic deposits. If the placental sections are too large to fit in the cassette, they will need to be divided. Additional representative sections of significant lesions or differences in villous character are also taken. En face blocks of the basal plate may be useful for evaluating maternal vasculature. It is not necessary to section every infarct, hemorrhagic lesion, and so forth, as long as they are clearly identifiable grossly and adequately described. Blocking can be done by a trained technician.

   The specific type of fixation, processing, cutting, and staining may greatly alter the histology of the placental villous tissue. This is particularly important in the assessment of villous structure and maturation. Anyone looking at even a few placentas needs to become familiar with the appearance of villous tissue at different points in gestation as prepared in their histology lab.

REPORTS

For reports, the original gross form can incorporate the microscopic exam and diagnoses or the gross data can be transferred to a second sheet (Appendix A-2). Such forms can serve as the actual report, or be the basis of a master which allows rapid typing of reports.

2
BASIC PLACENTAL ANATOMY AND DEVELOPMENT

Some appreciation of placental development is necessary to understand its examination and pathology. While the placenta shows extensive growth and histologic change in the second and third trimesters, the basic gross morphology is established early in pregnancy, before the end of the first trimester.

EARLY DEVELOPMENT

Trophoblastic tissue is the major component of the placenta. By 4 to 5 days after fertilization, trophoblasts differentiate from the external cells of the morula as it becomes a blastocyst. The trophoblastic cells proliferate rapidly and surround the inner cell mass, covering the entire surface of the blastocyst. Attachment to the endometrial surface and implantation occur at 5 to 6 days. Implantation is interstitial and the blastocyst becomes totally embedded in the endometrium. The endometrial stroma undergoes decidual change. The decidua between the blastocyst and myometrium is the decidua basalis, that covering the surface defect is the decidua capsularis, and that lining the rest of the uterus is the decidua parietalis. Usually implantation occurs in the upper portion of the uterus. As the developing conception grows, it protrudes into the endometrial cavity. At first the entire gestational sac is covered by chorionic villi (Figure 2-1). As the sac enlarges, its surface thins, forming the peripheral membranes which are composed of decidua capsularis, atrophied chorion, and amnion. The definitive placenta is left at the base (Figures 2-2 and 2-3). With continued growth of the conception there is apposition of the membranes with the decidua vera of the opposite side of the uterus, but no true fusion.

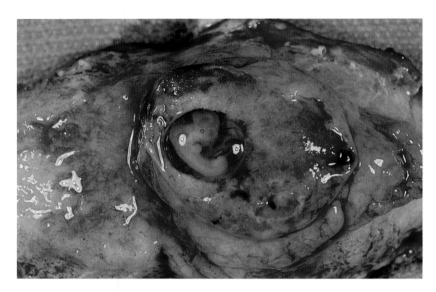

Figure 2-1. This embryo of 6 developmental weeks was removed *in situ* during a hysterectomy for cervical carcinoma. The decidua has been partially removed to reveal the chorionic villi which cover the entire early gestational sac. Part of the chorion has also been dissected showing the amniotic sac containing the embryo.

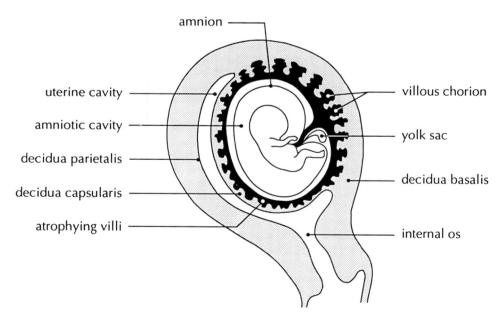

Figure 2-2. The embryo lies within the chorionic and amniotic sacs. Note the yolk sac between them. The capsular chorionic villi associated with the evolving peripheral membranes are undergoing atrophy creating the discoid placenta at the base into which the cord inserts.

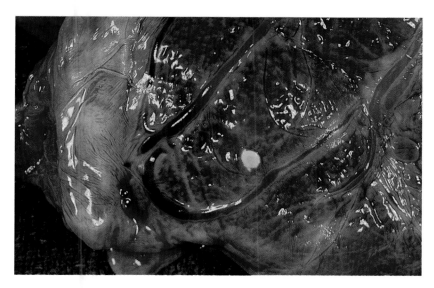

Figure 2-3.   The yellow 4-mm nodule is the calcified remnant of the yolk sac. It lies free under the amnion and above the chorion. These are quite commonly found in normal term placentas and are usually located near the edge of the placenta or in the membranes.

TROPHOBLAST

By the time of implantation, the trophoblast has differentiated into central uninucleate cytotrophoblast and peripheral multinucleated syncytiotrophoblast. The latter is nonmitotic and grows through fusion and incorporation of cytotrophoblast nuclei. The cytotrophoblast retains the capacity for mitosis throughout gestation, but has little functional differentiation compared to the active syncytiotrophoblast. A third type of trophoblastic cell, the uninucleate "intermediate" trophoblast, is predominantly involved in invasion of the placental bed and maternal blood vessels.

CIRCULATION

The feto-placental circulation begins at about 9 days when lacunae form in the syncytial trophoblast. By days 10 to 12 these link with maternal blood vessels which have been eroded by trophoblastic invasion. The primary fetal chorionic villi have formed by 14 days and consist of cords of cytotrophoblast covered by syncytial trophoblast. Within a day or so there is invasion of avascular extraembryonic mesenchyme from the embryonic body stalk into these columns forming secondary villi. Capillaries develop within the villous stroma and form networks by 20 days (tertiary villi). These vessels communicate with the fetus through vessels differentiating from the chorion and the connecting stalk, the large surface vessels and umbilical cord. The circulation is functional by the end of the third week. The placental tissue grows through branching of the villous tree. Primary stem villi break up below the chorionic plate to form the secondary and tertiary stem villi and finally the terminal villi. "Anchoring" villi are present at the base of the placenta.

PLACENTA ACCRETA

Invasion of the placenta into the uterine wall should stop before the myometrium is reached, with a layer of decidual tissue separating the anchoring villi from the muscle. If such limitation does not occur the placenta will be abnormally adherent and may extend into the uterine wall. Placenta acreta, increta or percreta results if there is invasion to, into, or through the myometrium respectively. These processes often occur in the setting of multiple previous cesarean sections or other uterine scarring. Destruction of the endometrium hampers formation of the decidua which appears to limit placen-

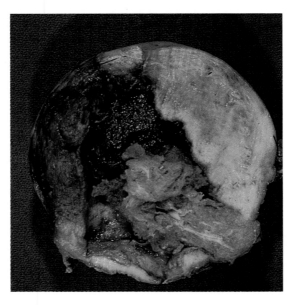

Figure 2-4. This fixed postpartum hysterectomy specimen reveals retained pale placental tissue invading focally nearly through the wall of the uterus, with thinning to less than 1 mm of serosal tissue (placenta increta).

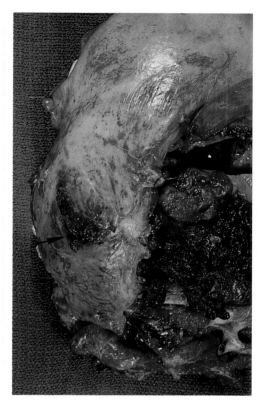

Figure 2-5.   This uterus still contains the bulk of the invasive placenta, which creates the bluish hue in the thinned lower uterine portion on the left. Focally the placental tissue has perforated the myometrium (*arrow*). An unsutured vertical cesarean section incision is present.

tal growth. It is usually not possible to make the diagnosis of accreta on a delivered placenta or curettings, and this process can often only be identified in hysterectomy specimens (Figures 2-4, 2-5, and 2-6).

PLACENTA PREVIA

Placenta previa arises when implantation occurs very low in the uterus and the placenta covers the cervix. This is often difficult to confirm on placental examination. If delivery was vaginal, finding the point of membrane rupture near the placental edge suggests marginal previa. Most complete previas are delivered by cesarean section. An area of old hemorrhage on the maternal

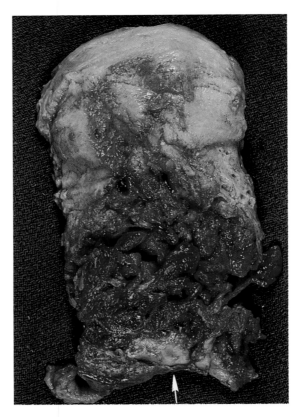

Figure 2-6. An opened uterus shows extensively invasive adherent placental tissue in the lower segment. Old clot (*arrow*) overlies the cervical os. Thus this was a placenta previa that had partially separated as well as an increta. Acreta, previa, and placental separation are frequently associated.

surface corresponding to the area of the cervical os may be present (Figure 2-7).

PLACENTAL SHAPE

The shape of the placenta is quite variable. Generally it is round to ovoid, and about 18–20 cm diameter by 1.5–2.5 cm thick at term. Failure of atrophy of capsular villi leads to succenturiate lobes (Figure 2-8). Bilobate placentas result from uterine sulcal implantation (Figure 2-9), while unusually shaped often multilobate placentas may be due to uterine cavity abnormalities (Figure 2-10). A diffuse thin placenta with little free membrane is known as a placenta membranacea. This may represent a shallow implantation with persistence of virtually all the peripheral villi.

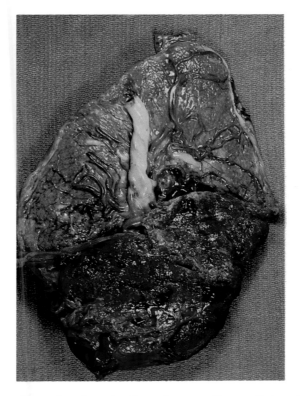

Figure 2-7. Implantation low in the uterus will result in placenta previa. Such pregnancies are almost invariably delivered by cesarean section. This near term placenta with complete placenta previa recapitulates the shape of the lower portion of the uterus, being folded back on itself at the cervix. There is brown, old hemorrhage in the area of the os due to placental separation.

PLACENTAL MATURATION

The gross morphology of the placenta is essentially established before the end of the first trimester, and further change is largely limited to growth and histologic maturation of villi. Normal maturation of villi entails several features. There is progressive diminution in villous size and stromal content and an increasing proportion of the villus is composed of blood vessels. The syncytiotrophoblast nuclei become aggregated into "knots," and their cell cytoplasm thins overlying vessels forming vasculosyncytial membranes. The originally very prominent cytotrophoblastic layer disappears and by term few cytotrophoblasts are recognized on light microscopy, although still present on electron microscopy (Figure 2-11).

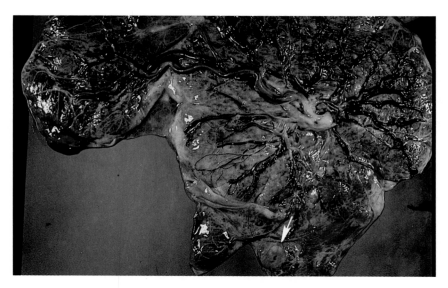

Figure 2-8. Succenturiate lobes are formed if some of the capsular villous tissue fails to atrophy during development. Such tissue can potentially be left behind at delivery leading to bleeding from retained placenta. These are usually connected to the main placental mass by velamentous vessels which can be damaged. Succenturiate lobes often become atrophic and fibrinous. This slightly immature placenta shows four such lobes, one large and three small. One of the latter is yellow and atrophic (*arrow*).

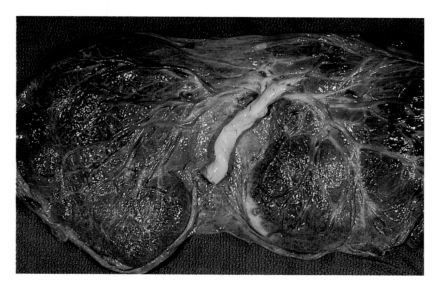

Figure 2-9. This mature bilobate placenta has two distinct lobes of roughly equal proportions. The umbilical cord inserts between them, into the membranes. Although this resembles a placenta with a large succenturiate lobe, this configuration probably arises through a different mechanism. Implantation in a lateral uterine sulcus leads to growth along the anterior and posterior walls.

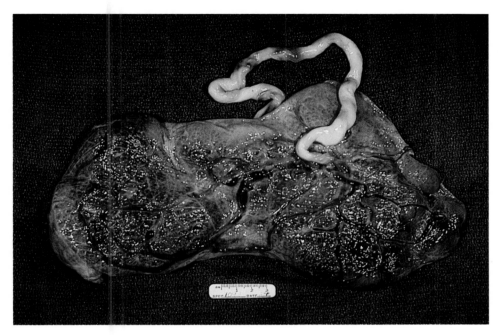

Figure 2-10. An unusual uterine shape, scarring, or intracavitary lesions may be reflected in the placental outline. Such abnormalities impede placental growth in certain areas and the placenta enlarges in the regions around them. This large irregular placenta has incomplete extra lobes suggesting an abnormal uterine cavity. Note also the hemolytic coloration, best seen in the cord and peripheral membranes. This usually results from improper storage temperature, or exposure to agents such as betadine.

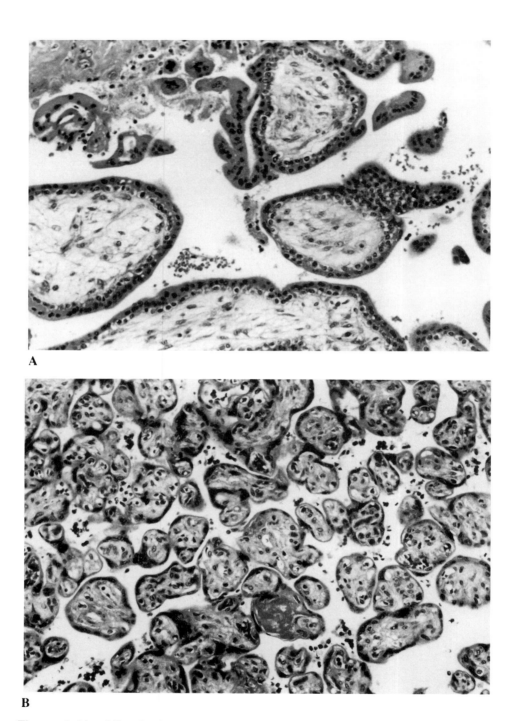

Figure 2-11. Histologic maturation of villi. (a) Very early first trimester villi show abundant stroma without vessels. Two layers of trophoblast are present, with no syncytial knots. (b) Term chorionic villi show little stroma and numerous blood vessels. Only syncytial trophoblast is visible on the surface with numerous knots.

3
UMBILICAL CORD

The umbilical cord is the lifeline of the fetus. Complete cord occlusion often leads to fetal demise while intermittent obstruction has been associated with intrauterine brain damage. Cord compression and vasospasm are important factors in fetal distress. Careful umbilical cord examination often reveals significant lesions which may be associated with these processes.

DEVELOPMENT

The umbilical cord forms in the region of the body stalk where the embryo is attached to the chorion. This area contains the allantois, evolving umbilical arteries and vein, omphalomesenteric duct, and vitelline vessels. The expanding amnion surrounds these structures and eventually covers the umbilical cord. Eventually most of the embryonic elements as well as the right umbilical vein disappear, leaving two arteries and one vein (Figure 3-1). Embryologic remnants are common in the cord, but are usually seen only on histology. Allantoic remnants show a transitional-type epithelium and occur most often near the fetal end, between the arteries. Omphalomesenteric remnants may be ductal, lined by gastrointestinal epithelium, or vascular (Figure 3-2). The spiral twisting of the cord is established early in development (Figures 3-3, 3-4, and 3-5).

LENGTH

One of the most obvious features of the umbilical cord is the length. It increases throughout gestation, although the growth rate slows in the third trimester. Fetal activity and stretch on the cord are major factors determining length. Normal tables have been developed (Appendices B-4 and B-5). Both

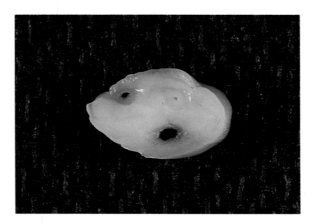

Figure 3-1. A normal three-vessel cord contains two arteries and one vein. The arteries are often more contracted than the vein, but it is not always possible to identify the type of vessel grossly. Most embryologic remnants are too small to be seen by eye.

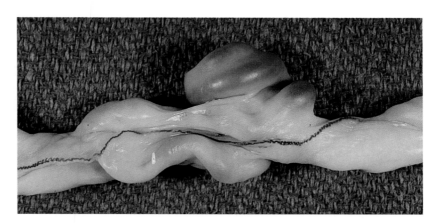

Figure 3-2. The dilated blue area is a "false knot" which represents a varicosity of an umbilical vessel. These are of no clinical significance, and are not prone to thrombosis or hemorrhage. The small zigzag vessel on the cord surface is a vitelline vascular remnant. Histologically, these have no muscular wall. They may be multiple suggesting hemangiomas.

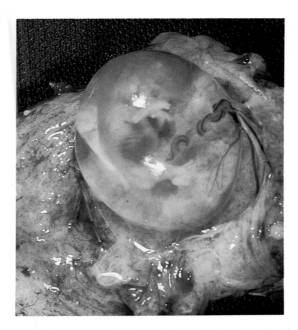

Figure 3-3. Umbilical cord twist is established early in development, as shown in this 10-week gestation. It usually twists in a left or counterclockwise direction (7:1). The reason for this is unclear but is not related to handedness.

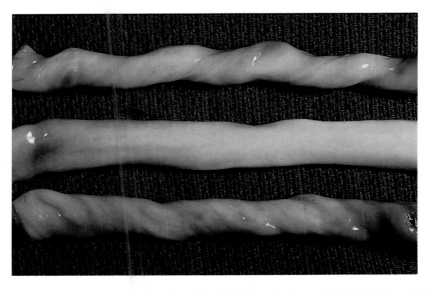

Figure 3-4. Umbilical cords showing left (*top*), absent (*middle*), and right (*bottom*) twists. Occasionally cords show two patterns. Infants whose cords lack a twist exhibit more perinatal morbidity. Cords missing one umbilical artery are also more frequently untwisted. No other correlations with fetal outcome have been identified.

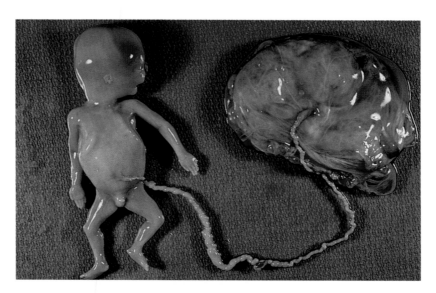

Figure 3-5. This midtrimester fetal demise shows an excessively long and twisted cord. Markedly twisted cords may be associated with fetal compromise or death. Such excessive twisting is not a postmortem artifact, and is seen throughout gestation. No other cause of fetal death was discerned on complete autopsy with karyotype. Isolated areas of true cord torsion and stricture also occur, particularly near the fetal body wall.

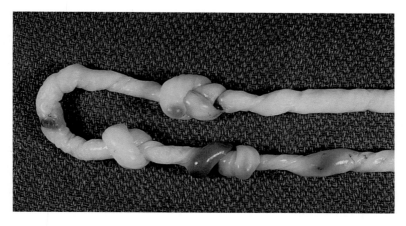

Figure 3-6. Knots and entanglements are common. Although the majority are not associated with problems, they do occasionally cause fetal distress and death. Knots should be carefully examined for the presence of differential congestion and/or thrombosis which suggest that the obstruction was functionally significant. These complicated knots occurred in a 31-week premature infant. There is slight congestion, but no thrombosis was noted.

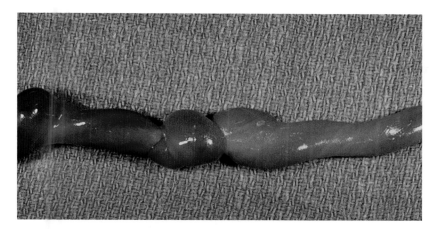

Figure 3-7. In fatal cord compressions, flow in the vein has usually been compromised, leading to congestion on the placental side (left). Such was the case in this intrauterine demise. One should be cautious in attributing a fetal death to a cord problem particularly if such secondary changes are absent. Entanglement can occur after fetal demise and the apparent cord problem may be incidental to the true cause of death.

abnormally long and short cords have significant clinical correlates. Long cords (>75 cm) are well associated with knots and fetal entanglements, and may correlate with later hyperactivity (Figures 3-6, 3-7, and 3-8). Thrombosis in cord vessel is an important sign of true obstruction (Figure 3-9). A minimum cord length of 32 cm is thought necessary for normal vaginal delivery, and undue traction can cause fetal distress, cord tearing, and possibly placental separation (Figures 3-10 and 3-11). Short cords are known to occur in disorders with decreased fetal movement (oligohydramnios, arthrogryposis). They are also associated with poor neurologic development. This suggests the associated infants may have had longstanding *in utero* problems compromising fetal mobility. Because of these associations, it is extremely important to measure the entire cord length, including that left on the baby or taken for cord gases. Ideally this is done in the delivery room.

Premature infants tend to have thicker umbilical cords than more mature babies, while cord substance is often lacking in growth retardation. Edema of the cord can be impressive, and is inconsistently seen in a variety of pathologic states (Figure 3-12).

INSERTION

The insertion of the cord into the placental disk can show a variety of abnormal configurations (Figures 3-13 to 3-21). The site may be into the placental substance or into membranes. The position of insertion is due to the plane

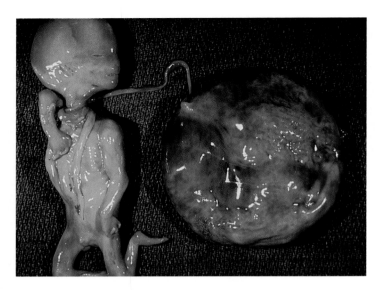

Figure 3-8. This midtrimester loss was thought to be due to true cord entanglement and occlusion. A complete autopsy including cytogenetics failed to reveal other significant pathology.

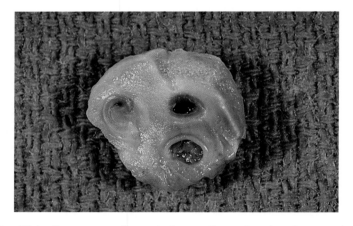

Figure 3-9. This three-vessel cord shows thrombosis of one artery. An occlusive thrombus in one umbilical artery can occur without fetal problems because of normal vascular anastomoses between the two arteries. The cord substance is discolored from leaking blood pigments. Thrombosis of a cord vessel will lead to necrosis of the wall as blood flow is its only nutrient source.

Umbilical Cord

25

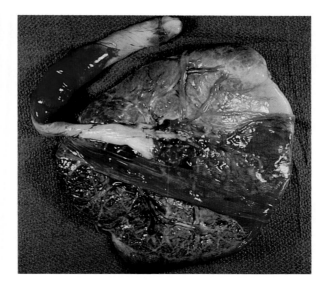

Figure 3-10. Many cord hemorrhages are artifactual, associated with clamping. This true hematoma, which enlarged the cord to 2 cm in diameter, did not show clamp marks. There was fetal distress in labor. Disruption of the vein was noted histologically along with very early thrombosis. Only 22 cm of cord was received with the placenta.

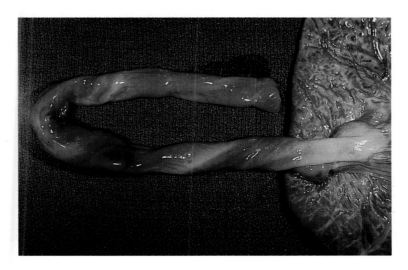

Figure 3-11. This hemorrhage occurred in a short cord with a complete length of 32 cm. The arterial hematoma compressed the umbilical vein and led to fetal demise. Early thrombosis was present. As in Figure 3-9 localized hemolytic discoloration of the cord substance is visible.

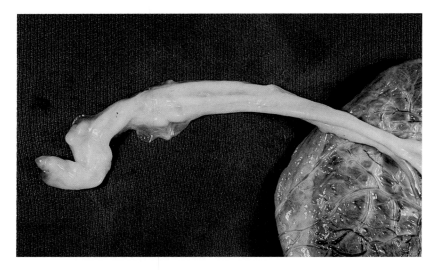

Figure 3-12. Marked edema is present in this umbilical cord. The vessels become cordlike strands within the very loose Wharton's jelly. Such edema may be associated with a variety of perinatal diseases including infection, preeclampsia, and hemorrhage. Prematurity and stillbirth are more common.

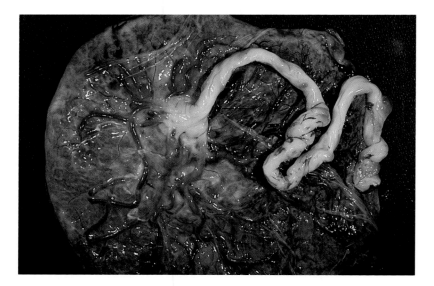

Figure 3-13. Most placentas will have a cord insertion in the center or slightly eccentric in the disk, the latter shown here. The surface vessels disperse from the cord in a relatively even circumferential manner. Even when the cord has been torn from the placenta, examining the distribution of surface blood vessels often reveals the site of insertion.

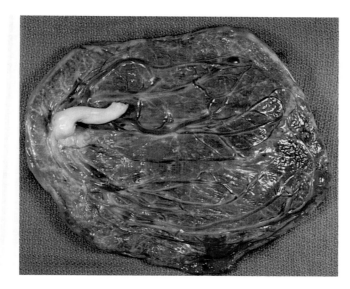

Figure 3-14. This cord inserts close, but not quite at the margin of the placenta. The vessels splay largely unidirectionally. Such a vascular distribution is found in 38% of placentas and is likely somewhat less effective in perfusion of the fetus.

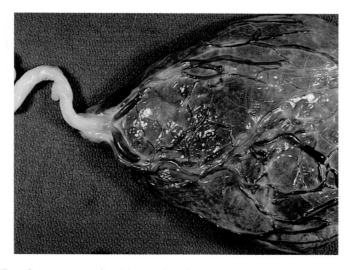

Figure 3-15. A true marginal insertion is present (Battledore placenta). Babies with such cords are slightly smaller on average, as are those with true velamentous insertions. Vessels in the membranes adjacent to marginal cord insertions are common. Marginal and velamentous cords may be less mobile and more prone to compromise.

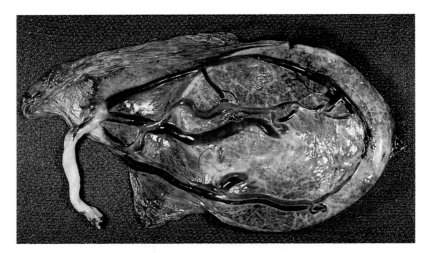

Figure 3-16. Insertion of the cord into the free membranes occurs in 1% of deliveries and is called a velamentous insertion. The distance from the placental edge to the cord should be measured, and the vessels carefully examined for their integrity. As with many very peripheral insertions, there is a paucity of fetal surface vessel ramifications. This may contribute to the associated growth retardation.

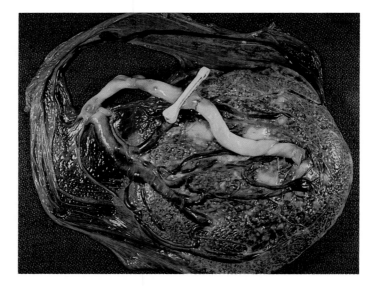

Figure 3-17. Despite the close proximity of the cord insertion and velamentous vessels to the site of membrane rupture in this vaginal delivery, no vascular disruption occurred. Vessels overlying the cervical os (vasa previa) are at the greatest risk of tearing, which results in catastrophic fetal blood loss. Velamentous vessels may also be prone to compression during labor.

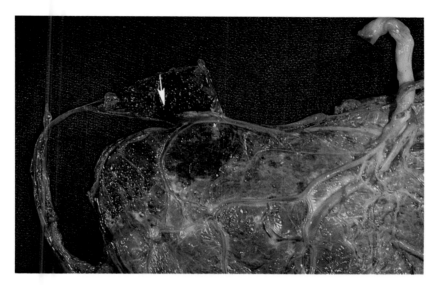

Figure 3-18. Rupture of a velamentous vessel occurred in this case (*arrow*). Maternal history and neonatal anemia indicated this had happened during labor. The infant survived. Vessels may also be torn after the infant has been born, during the delivery of the placenta. While this will be of no clinical significance, it should be noted since complete historical information may not be available at the time of placental examination.

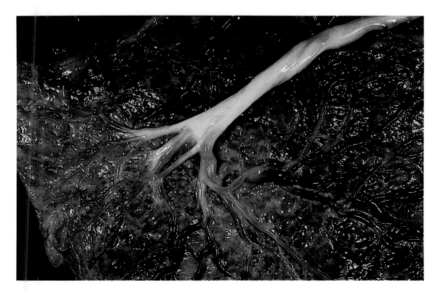

Figure 3-19. This cord divides into vessels which lose their protective covering of Wharton's jelly above the surface of the placenta. Such furcate insertions will have the risks attendant to velamentous vessels.

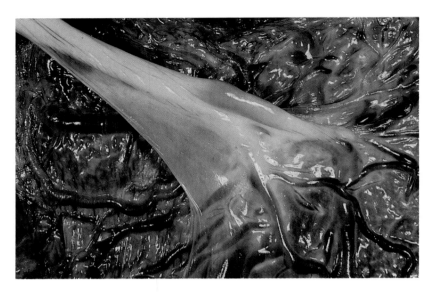

Figure 3-20. At times the cord is partially encased by a fold of amnion at its placental end, a "chorda" or amniotic web. These can extend for several centimeters up the cord and be loose or relatively tight, binding the cord to the fetal surface of the placenta.

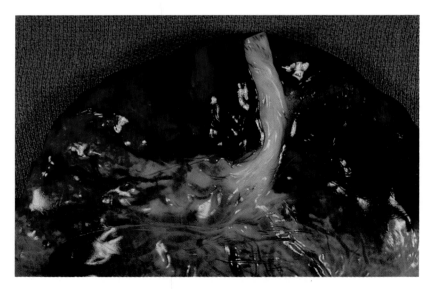

Figure 3-21. A long tight amniotic web is present. Such webs may limit the mobility of the cord, potentially compromising blood flow. This placenta also shows subamniotic hemorrhage. Although bleeding from vessels between the amnion and chorion is likely an artifact arising during placental delivery, it attests to the stress from such webs.

of implantation of the conception and/or differential placental growth from uterine conditions. Placentas with velamentous vessels are particularly important to evaluate and document, since such vessels can be associated with compression or rupture. Rupture may cause extremely rapid fetal exsanguination (Figure 3-18).

SINGLE UMBILICAL ARTERY

The absence of one umbilical artery is a common anomaly, occurring in about 1% of deliveries (Figure 3-22). It is more frequently seen with twins and velamentous cord insertions. About 20% of infants missing one artery will have other major congenital anomalies which may involve any organ system. Many are of chromosomal etiology. The abnormalities are generally apparent in the neonatal period, except for the increased incidence of inguinal hernias. The "nonmalformed" infants missing one umbilical artery are slightly growth-retarded overall and have increased perinatal mortality. Cord accidents have been unusually frequent in this group.

INFECTION

The cord inflammation seen with most ascending membranous infections (see page 46) is not recognizable grossly. Candida, however, shows characteristic microabscesses on the cord surface (Figures 3-23, 3-24, and 3-25). This infection may cause a rash on the infant at birth. It is more likely to cause sepsis in premature infants. The "barber-pole" configuration of chronic necrotizing funisitis is felt to represent a chronic and sometimes healed intrauterine infection with organisms of low virulence (Figures 3-26 and 3-27).

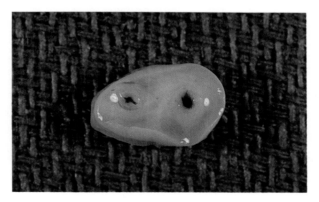

Figure 3-22. An umbilical cord with a single umbilical artery shows only two vascular lumens. Normally the two arteries may fuse in the last few centimeters of cord above the fetal surface, thus multiple cuts more distal should be made to confirm this finding.

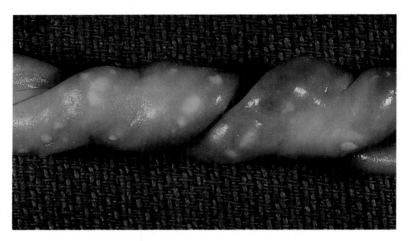

Figure 3-23. Scattered yellow to white 2–3 mm plaques on the cord are virtually pathognomonic of *Candida* funisitis. They are not seen elsewhere on the placental membranes.

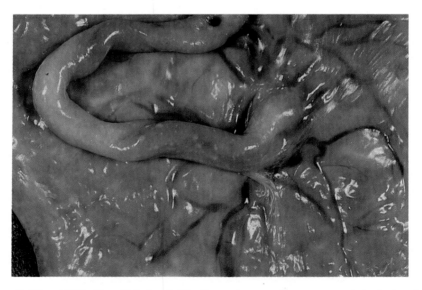

Figure 3-24. With *Candida* funisitis there is usually an associated chorioamnionitis. This caused the severe yellow-green discoloration of the fetal surface. Cord lesions can also be seen here.

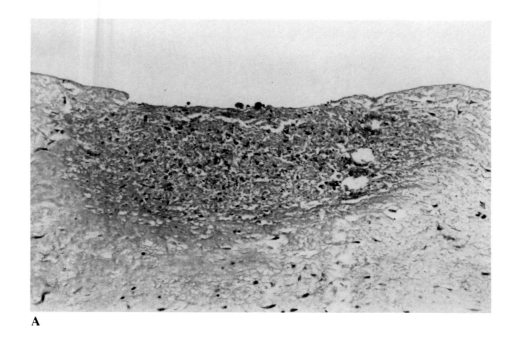

A

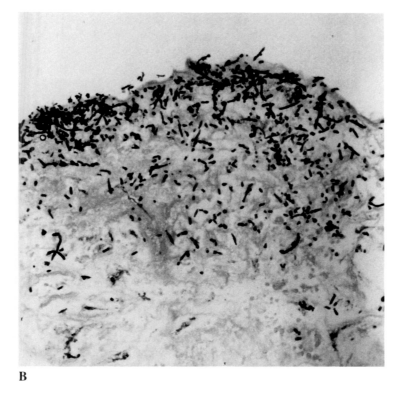

B

Figure 3-25. (a) Histologically the cord in *Candida* funisitis shows microab-scesses lying just under the surface. These are filled with necrotic debris in which it is difficult to identify organisms. (b) Numerous fungal pseudohyphae and yeasts are present on methenamine silver stain.

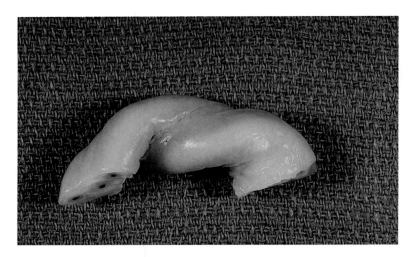

Figure 3-26. Necrotizing funisitis represents a chronic inflammatory process in the umbilical cord, apparently infectious in origin. "Barber-pole"
striping of the cord is seen. The calcification surrounding the vessels leads
to an extremely rigid cord.

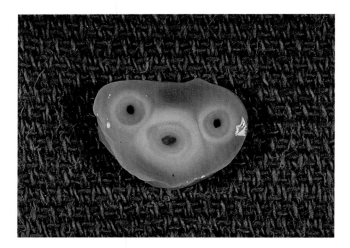

Figure 3-27. Cross section of a cord with necrotizing funisitis shows white
bands suggesting diffusion rings surrounding each of the three vessels.
These are composed of necrotic inflammatory cells and calcium.

4
FETAL MEMBRANES AND SURFACE

LAYERS

The peripheral membranes and fetal placental surface are continuous, and most processes affect the entire area. The layer of membrane closest to the fetus is amnion. Adjacent is chorion, minimal on the peripheral membranes and more extensive on the disk. There is close proximity of the surface membranes to the maternal blood of the intervillous space, while the peripheral membranes abut the decidua and its blood vessels. This relationship permits maternal cells access to the membranes. Deposits from the maternal circulation are common beneath the fetal surface. As pregnancy progresses, the amount of such fibrin and thrombotic material generally increases (Figures 4-1 and 4-2). The quantity of subchorionic fibrin has been associated with fetal activity and eventual outcome.

SUBCHORIONIC HEMORRHAGE

Thick layers of subchorionic hemorrhage can be associated with chronic bleeding and prematurity (Figures 4-3 and 4-4). Large nodular subchorionic hematomas, sometimes called ''Breus moles,'' are seen in both liveborns and spontaneous abortions. Such hemorrhages are difficult to identify on ultrasound and may be confused with other processes such as chorangiomas. Induced abortions (e.g., prostaglandin) usually have extensive fresh subchorionic hemorrhage (Figure 4-5).

EXTRACHORIAL PLACENTATION

The membranes normally insert at the peripheral margin of the villous tissue which is usually the outer limit of the vascular plate. Extrachorial placen-

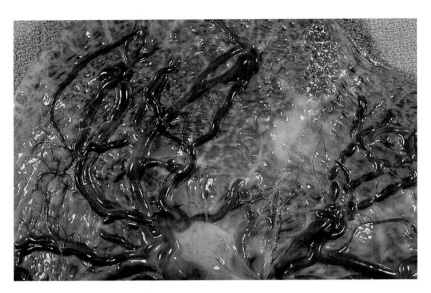

Figure 4-1. Subchorionic fibrin tends to increase with gestational age, although it is quite variable. This is often a striking feature of the fetal surface, and may be quite dense, as seen in this term placenta. When possible, areas with thick fibrin should be avoided for histologic sections and the more transparent regions of the surface sampled. Inflammatory processes are often masked in areas with thick fibrin.

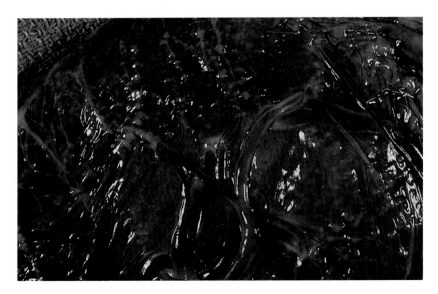

Figure 4-2. An immature placenta shows minimal subchorionic fibrin, leading to the deep blue surface coloration commonly seen.

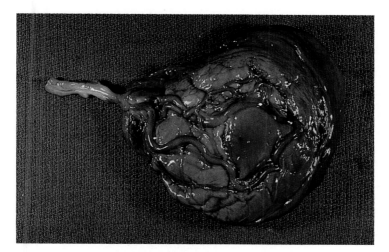

Figure 4-3. Extensive thick clot and hemorrhage undermine the fetal surface in this case, a change which may be found as early as midtrimester. The membranes are discolored from hemosiderin pigment, and the amniotic fluid may be thick and brown. Placentas such as this are sometimes called "Breus moles." This placenta also shows a velamentous insertion of the umbilical cord.

tation exists when villous tissue extends outward beyond the vascular plate. This takes two forms, circummargination and circumvallation (Figure 4-6). In the former there is a small ridge of fibrin where the membranes contact the extended placental surface (Figure 4-7), while in circumvallation there is a redundant, doubled-back membrane fold with enclosed old hemorrhage at the point of membrane insertion (Figures 4-8 and 4-9). Circummargination is not believed to lead to clinical problems, but prematurity and chronic bleeding are associated with circumvallation. The origin of extrachorial placentation is unclear. Suggestions include abnormal implantation, secondary growth lines, marginal separation, and loss of amniotic fluid pressure.

AMNION NODOSUM/SQUAMOUS METAPLASIA

Nodularity of the amnion represents either amnion nodosum or squamous metaplasia. These are important to distinguish. Squamous metaplasia is a normal variant (Figure 4-10), while amnion nodosum is strongly associated with profound, longstanding oligohydramnios, a setting in which pulmonary hypoplasia commonly develops (Figures 4-11, 4-12, and 4-13).

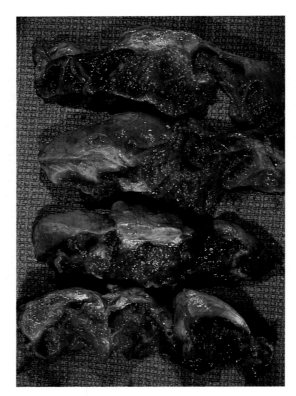

Figure 4-4. Cross sections of a placenta similar to that in Figure 4-3 better show the subchorionic extension of the clot and separation of the villous tissue from the fetal surface. Such placentas can be associated with early oligohydramnios, bleeding, elevated α-fetoprotein, and preterm delivery of small, nonmalformed infants, who sometimes have pulmonary hypoplasia. The etiology of this process is unknown, but there may be a risk of recurrence.

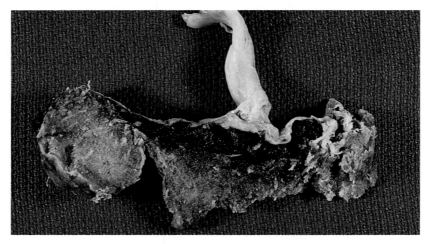

Figure 4-5. Cross section of an immature placenta shows extensive fresh hemorrhage under the chorionic surface. This is usual when delivery has been induced by prostaglandins. It also occurs with saline terminations.

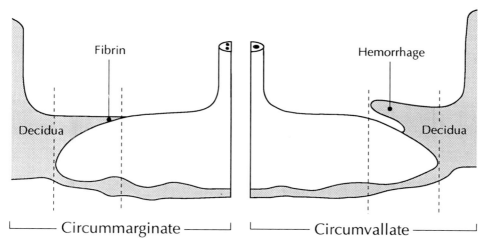

Figure 4-6. Extrachorial placentation is displayed schematically with the extrachorial portion enclosed by dotted lines. The right cross section shows the redundant membrane fold characteristic of circumvallation. This frequently contains old hemorrhage continuous with the decidua. Such changes are absent in circummargination (left) in which the membranes are flat with a small deposit of fibrin.

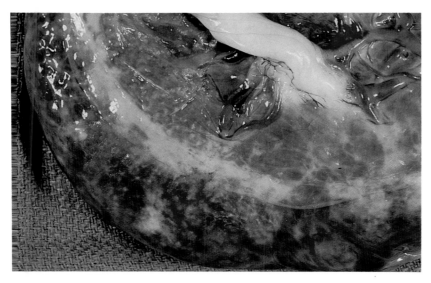

Figure 4-7. Circummarginate ring on a term placenta shows a thin rim of fibrin where the vascular plate abuts the extension of the placental tissue. The surface is flat and there is no hemorrhage at the margin. Circummargination may involve all or only part of the placental circumference, and the width of the extension varies from about 1 to >10 cm. Most believe there are no pathologic sequelae from this process, which may represent a secondary growth line.

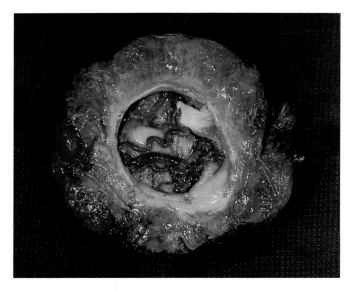

Figure 4-8. This circumvallate placenta shows a complete circumferential fold of membranes where the vascular plate ends. Hemorrhage often occurs in this marginal area, and these placentas are frequently thicker than usual. The process may be total or partial. Circumvallation, whose etiology is unknown, is associated with preterm bleeding and early delivery.

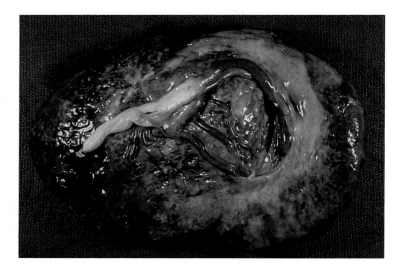

Figure 4-9. This placenta incorporates features of both circumvallation and circummargination, which is not unusual. It is extremely thick with circumferential extension of placental tissue beyond the plate. A small fold of membrane is present at 5 o'clock. Old hemorrhage is present at the rim for nearly half the circumference. There is also a paucity of surface vessels. Such extensive reduction in the fetal surface vasculature could affect fetal perfusion.

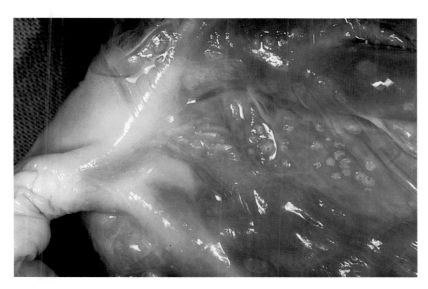

Figure 4-10. Squamous metaplasia is an incidental change in the amnion. The normally cuboidal epithelium becomes nonkeratinizing squamous type. This change is most commonly seen near the cord insertion where it appears as small, dull, white plaques which are not readily removed with scraping.

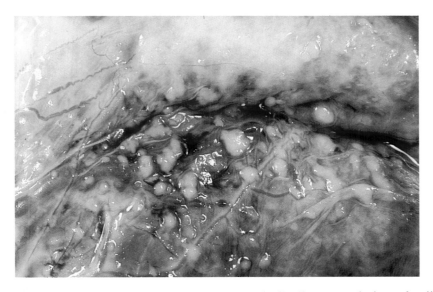

Figure 4-11. Amnion nodosum is a pathologic finding, consisting of yellow-white nodules of hair and squames pressed onto the fetal surface. These nodules are not adherent and can be easily removed. They may be found all over the placental surface and membranes. Amnion nodosum occurs in the setting of severe oligohydramnios, and is a marker for its prior existence. Such infants often have pulmonary hypoplasia.

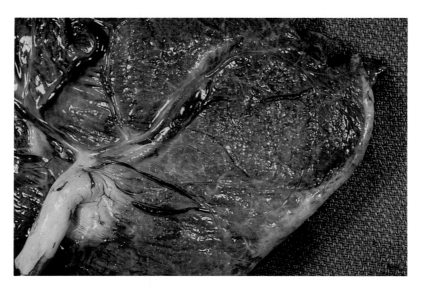

Figure 4-12. Another appearance of amnion nodosum is shown in this placenta which has a finely granular appearance over much of its surface. This is often much harder to recognize. The severity of amnion nodosum tends to be greater later in gestation, but is quite variable.

AMNIOTIC RUPTURE

Occasionally the amnion ruptures before delivery. The resulting bands of amnion can entrap and disrupt fetal tissues leading to defects including amputations, clefts, and constrictions (Figures 4-14 and 4-15). They may encircle the umbilical cord and cause fetal death. This process has a negligible risk of recurrence and placental examination can often make the diagnosis. Pregnancies in which the fetus develops outside the membranes, extramembranous gestations, also show characteristic placental changes (Figure 4-16). Oligohydramnios occurs with these lesions as the exposed chorion leads to altered amniotic fluid dynamics.

CYSTS

Cysts are frequently found on the surface of the term placenta (Figure 4-17). While most are only a few centimeters in diameter, they are occasionally much larger (Figure 4-18). Cysts tend to be seen when there is abundant placental fibrin deposition. Intermediate-type trophoblast ("X" cells) proliferates in such areas and becomes cystic. Cysts do not appear to have other

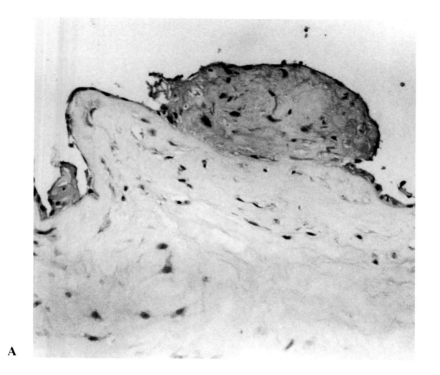

A

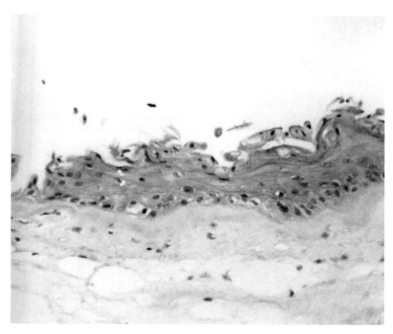

B

Figure 4-13. Histology of amnion nodosum compared to squamous meta-plasia. (a) In amnion nodosum nodules of hair, squames, and amorphous material are compressed on the surface, leading to destruction of the under-lying amniotic epithelium. (b) Squamous metaplasia shows a change in the cuboidal amniotic epithelium to a keratinizing squamous type.

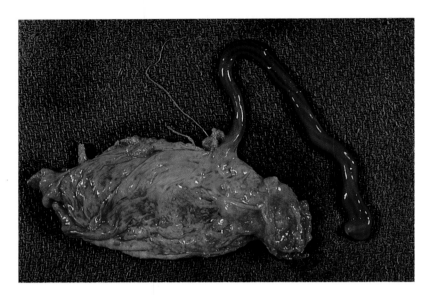

Figure 4-14. The strand of tissue attached to this immature, hemorrhagic placenta associated with a fetal demise is an amniotic band. Bands can be quite delicate and require careful examination to distinguish them from artifact. Chorion comprises the placental surface covering. Squames may be present on the surface chorion, similar to amnion nodosum.

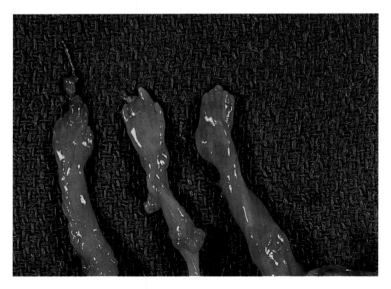

Figure 4-15. The macerated fetus associated with the placenta in Figure 4-14 was fragmented in delivery. Characteristic digital amputation defects of amniotic bands can still be visualized.

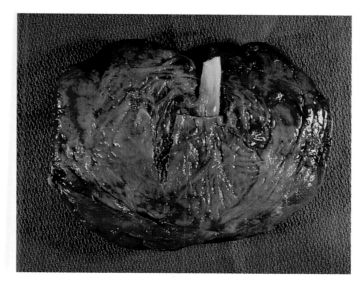

Figure 4-16. This placenta is from an extramembranous pregnancy in which the membranes ruptured before delivery. There is yellow-green discoloration from old hemorrhage. The membranes are everted and closely applied to the fetal surface. Squames were present on the chorionic surface.

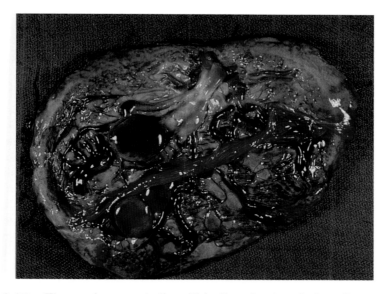

Figure 4-17. The surface cysts lie within the chorion, below the amnion, as can be seen near the bottom where the amnion has been reflected leaving the cysts intact. Hemorrhage may occur within these, as shown in the cyst by the cord insertion. There is abundant subchorionic fibrin.

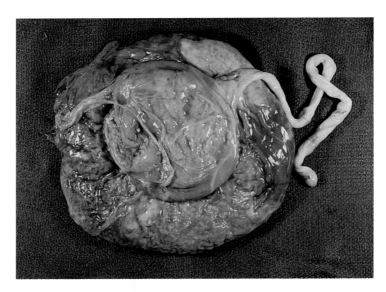

Figure 4-18. Surface cysts can become quite large, as shown here. Extensive old hemorrhage fills the lesion, which was worrisome on ultrasound. Despite the rather impressive appearance of such cysts, they have no known direct clinical consequences.

intrinsic significance. Similar lesions are seen within placental septae (Figure 5-35).

INFECTION

Color and translucency of the membranes are quite variable, depending on pigmentation, edema, cellular content, and amount of attached decidua (Figure 4-19). One of the most frequent causes of surface opacity is ascending infection with neutrophilic infiltration of the membranes, chorioamnionitis. This is the most common type of placental infection and is due to contamination of the amniotic fluid by organisms from the vaginal tract. The infectious process involves the surface and peripheral membranes, and infiltrates of inflammatory cells lead to the opacified appearance (Figures 4-20, 4-21, and 4-22). Frequently this process is clinically unsuspected. The usual agents are bacteria, although *Candida* and herpes simplex also infect in this manner. If sepsis occurs in the first few days of life, the placenta usually shows ascending infection. However, the vast majority (95%) of infants with chorioamnionitis do not become septic. There are strong indications that chorioamnionitis initiates a substantial portion of premature labor and premature rupture of the membranes. Such inflammation may also lead to fetal vascular reactivity and subsequent hypoxia.

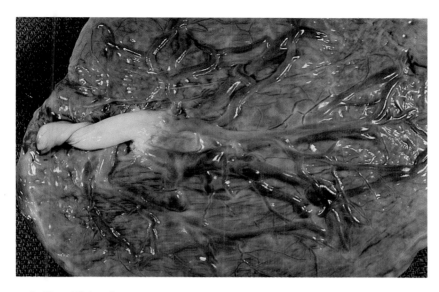

Figure 4-19. This placenta shows a mild degree of surface membrane opacity. While this often indicates ascending infection, membrane edema or remote meconium pigmentation may give a similar appearance. It is often difficult to be sure of the diagnosis grossly.

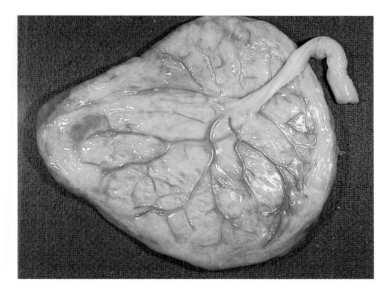

Figure 4-20. There is marked opacity of the fetal surface in this severely infected immature placenta. The slight yellow-green coloration is due to myeloperoxidase from the numerous neutrophils. Such placentas can be foul smelling, particularly in anaerobic infections, which occur commonly.

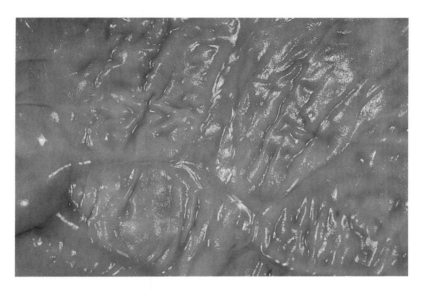

Figure 4-21. Another severely infected placenta shows prominent green coloration. There is obliteration of the surface vasculature, due in part to the fetal vasculitis associated with ascending infection. This can be a helpful gross feature to distinguish inflamed placentas.

MECONIUM

Meconium in the amniotic fluid commonly causes green discolored membranes in late gestation. An exposed placenta can have several gross appearances (Figures 4-23, 4-24, and 4-25). The time course of histologic meconium change is not clearly established. *In vitro* studies suggest meconium rapidly reaches macrophages in the amnion (one hour) (Figure 4-26) and is in the chorion within three hours. Whether this corresponds to the time course *in vivo* is unknown, but alterations almost certainly occur within hours, not days. The passage of meconium has long been taken as a sign of fetal stress. Current thinking regarding the significance of meconium in the amniotic fluid is less defined. Some, but not all, infants in distress pass meconium, and many infants with meconium have not had hypoxic events. A few pigmented macrophages in the membranes are common on careful examination of term placentas. The presence of substantial meconium in the amniotic fluid may, however, lead to umbilical vasoconstriction, and some severely meconium-stained cords show necrosis of peripheral vascular muscle cells. This latter finding is particularly associated with poor pregnancy outcome. All green placentas do not have meconium. Extensive old hemorrhage or severe ascending infection can lead to this coloration (Figures 4-16 and 4-21). These are important considerations in preterm pregnancies (less than 35 weeks) when passage of meconium is unlikely.

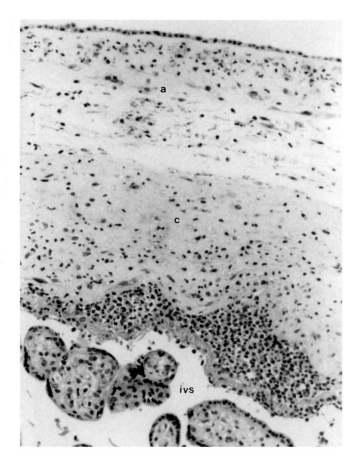

Figure 4-22.   Histology of chorioamnionitis reveals neutrophils from the maternal intervillous space (ivs) extending into the chorion (c) and amnion (a).

HEMORRHAGE

Red-brown thickenings and yellow areas mark old hemorrhages behind the membranes (Figures 4-27 and 4-28). These result from confined regions of hemorrhage in areas of decidual necrosis, and are usually of little consequence.

THROMBOSIS

The fetal surface vessels may show thrombosis or calcification, most commonly in a fetal vein (Figures 4-29 to 4-32). Sometimes thrombosis occurs with inflammation, meconium, or vascular obstruction, but many have no apparent causation. Calcification of vessel walls represents old thrombosis. Many thrombi histologically take the form of fibrinous plaques (Figure 4-33).

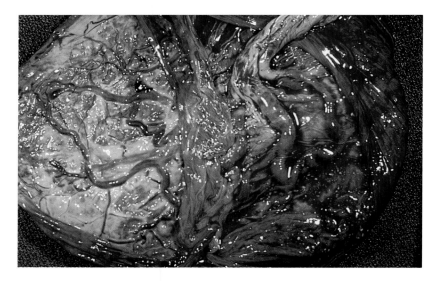

Figure 4-23. Fetal passage of meconium leads to green coloration of the placenta. This placenta shows very recent meconium, which sits on the amnion and does not stain the chorion revealed by reflection of the amnion on the left. Experimental studies suggest chorionic staining takes approximately 3 hours. Meconium has a variety of appearances. It may be thick or thin and color ranges from yellow to dark green.

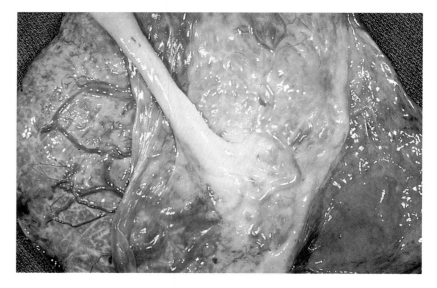

Figure 4-24. This meconium-stained placenta shows yellow-green coloration of the chorion, suggesting a longer duration of passage.

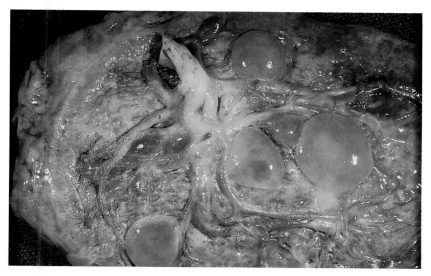

Figure 4-25. This mature placenta has a vaguely green color. This most likely represents more remote meconium passage and the surface is colored by pigment-laden macrophages. However, some placentas with such green coloration will be found to have ascending infection or iron deposition. Meconium alone does not lead to an inflammatory response, although it may predispose to infection and they are often seen together. Numerous cysts are also present here.

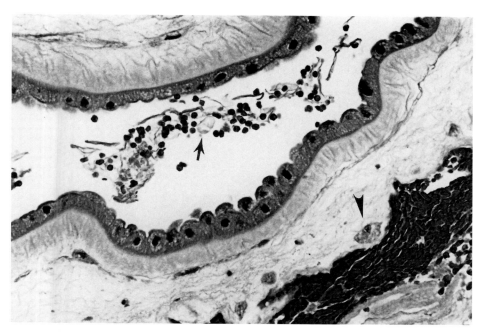

Figure 4-26. Histology of membranes stained with meconium reveals fresh, free meconium containing squames and hair (*arrow*) as well as vacuolated pigmented macrophages in the amniotic connective tissue (*arrowhead*). The pigment does not stain for iron. These changes may be as recent as 1 hour.

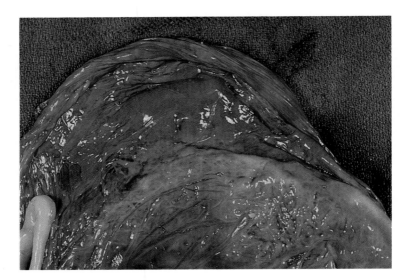

Figure 4-27. Brown or yellow discolorations on the membranes usually reflect old, retromembranous hemorrhages. While these may be associated with other hemorrhage in the placenta, they are frequently isolated. Such lesions are quite common. A clinical history of mild bleeding can sometimes be elicited.

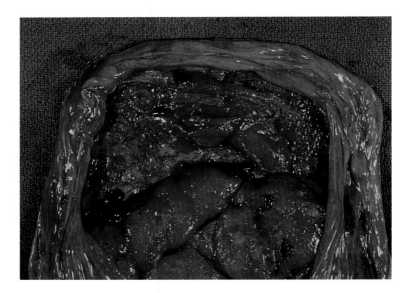

Figure 4-28. The maternal surface better shows the old brown-red clotted blood on the membranes.

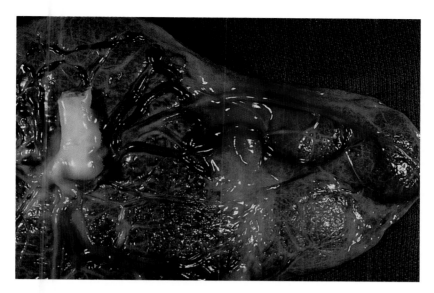

Figure 4-29. Two regions of tan and red thrombosed arteries and veins are present on the surface of this placenta. Hemolytic coloration of the surrounding membranes denotes these areas. One group connects to several succenturiate lobes. The vessels run through thinned placental tissue raising the possibility of obstruction as the etiology here. Another group, however, is present on the main disc. There was extensive associated villous change (Figure 5-28).

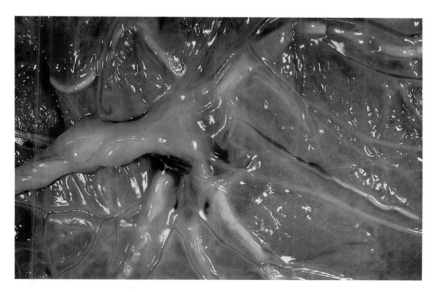

Figure 4-30. Thrombi and vascular calcifications are seen in veins on the fetal surface. Veins are the most common location for these changes. Since fetal arteries cross over veins, the vessels can be distinguished grossly. Identification is more difficult histologically. This pale, discolored placenta was associated with premature closure of the foramen ovale, hydrops, and intrauterine demise.

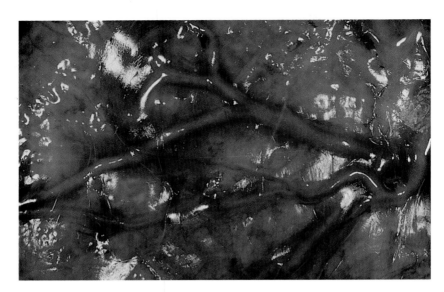

Figure 4-31. In this severely meconium-stained placenta, venous thrombosis can be identified. It is from a recent fetal demise who showed changes of fetal anoxia and massive meconium aspiration.

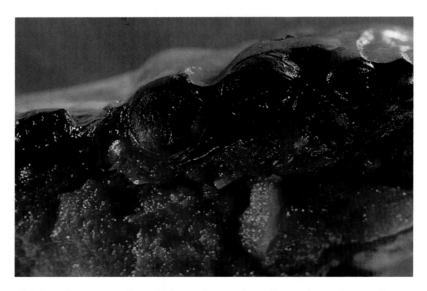

Figure 4-32. Cross-sectional view of a surface thrombus shows the granular nature. Often thrombi are not fully occlusive of the vessel, as is the case here.

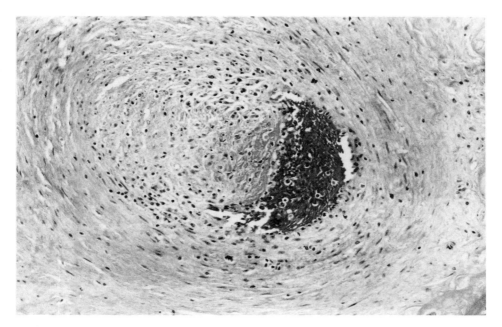

Figure 4-33. Histologic view of a partially occluded large fetal vessel shows fibrinous material on one side. The cellularity of the wall suggests that inflammation may have initiated this thrombosis.

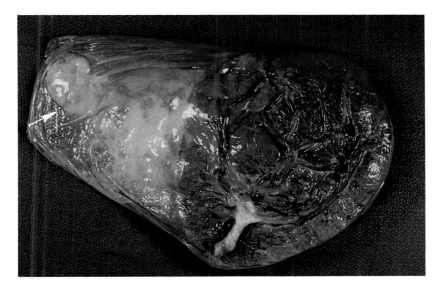

Figure 4-34. Careful examination of the membranes may reveal the presence of an atrophied twin (*arrow*). These are usually firm ovoid nodules with a smooth outline, as distinct from old hemorrhage or decidual necrosis. Examination of the dividing membranes revealed this to be a monochorionic twin. Size suggested 12 weeks gestation.

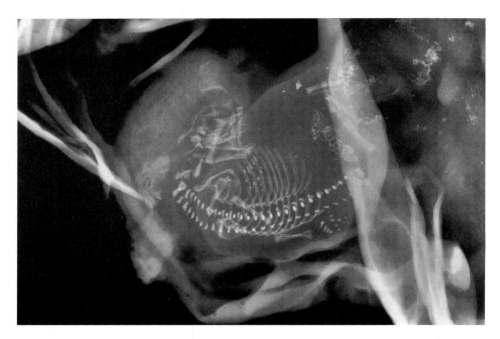

Figure 4-35. Specimen radiograph of Figure 4-34 shows the fetal nature of the nodule. Skeletal examination will reveal gestational age and some anomalies.

FETUS PAPYRACEOUS

In these times of assisted reproduction, it is important to identify lost pregnancies in multiple gestations. The recognition of long dead fetuses usually relies on the careful examination of the membranes, where they are commonly found. Some appear as fibrinous plaques, while others have a more recognizable form (Figures 4-34, 6-11, and 6-21). Zygosity can often be determined (see Chapter 6). X-rays may be useful for identification and dating (Figure 4-35).

5
LESIONS OF THE VILLOUS TISSUE

The villous tissue is examined from the maternal side both before and after transverse cuts have been made in the surface. While visual inspection is important, palpation of the placenta may be even more revealing of pathologic processes. Most grossly identified villous lesions show a diagnostic morphology. Many of the common abnormalities reflect the placental circulation (Figure 5-1), and aberrations in the fetal and maternal components can both be recognized.

CALCIFICATION

Calcification may be a striking feature of the maternal surface and villous tissue (Figure 5-2). The degree is quite variable and the etiology is unknown. Generally, calcification increases with gestational age. Even very large amounts have no recognized pathologic sequelae.

COLOR

The color of the villous tissue tends to darken with advancing gestational age. Color is largely determined by fetal hemoglobin content, thus immature infants who characteristically have lower hematocrits, have paler placentas than term infants (Figure 5-3). Unusual fetal vascular congestion or fetal blood loss will lead to dark or light villous color (Figure 5-4). Hydrops fetalis characteristically shows a very pale placenta (Figures 5-5, 5-6, and 5-7). There are many etiologies for hydrops including isoimmunization, infection, cytogenetic abnormalities, malformations, and metabolic disease. Some of these are readily diagnosed through placental histology.

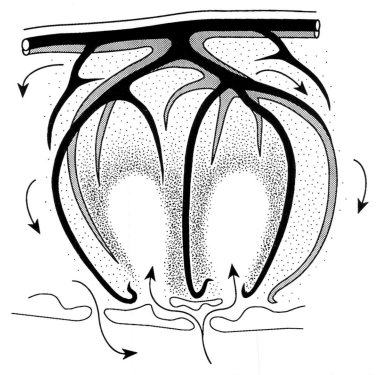

Figure 5-1. In this schematic of a placental district, maternal blood is shown being injected from altered decidual spiral arterioles (bottom) into the central intervillous space where it often leaves a "hole" (see Figure 5-4). The blood flows toward the fetal surface, and drains back passively to decidual veins. The midzone of the placenta is best perfused, with poorer flow at the base, under the fetal surface, and at the margins. The fetal arteries (*solid*) run over fetal veins (*hatched*) and both branch to capillaries at the villous level.

INFARCTS

True villous infarcts are quite common and usually distinctive on gross exam. These are villous regions that have lost their maternal blood supply and are based on the maternal surface (Figure 5-8). Infarcts are more solid than the adjacent tissue and appear granular from the remaining villous ghosts. Over time color changes from red to white (Figures 5-9 and 5-10). Infarction is common at margin, and a small (1-cm) lesion of this nature is usually insignificant (Figures 5-11 and 5-12). Central and large marginal infarcts suggest maternal vascular disease, particularly if they are extensive (Figure 5-13). Histologically, early infarcts show villous congestion and collapse with loss of the intervillous space, accounting for the gross firmness and red color.

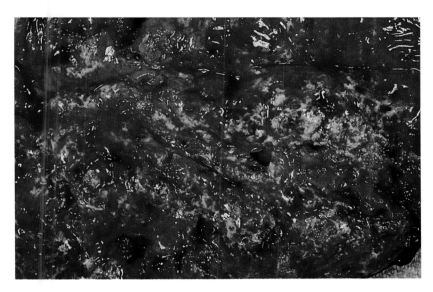

Figure 5-2. Yellow-white areas of abundant calcification can be seen on the maternal surface of this normal term placenta. It will also be present within the parenchyma, giving a gritty sensation and sound on cutting. Grossly visible calcification is quite variable, but tends to increase with advancing gestation. It is not associated with disease, even if large amounts are present.

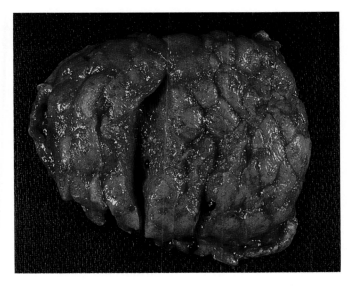

Figure 5-3. The floor and parenchyma of this normal immature (20-week) placenta show no calcification and are moderately pale. Color of the villous tissue is largely related to hemoglobin content. Thus mature placentas have a darker coloration than immature ones (compare with Figure 1-6).

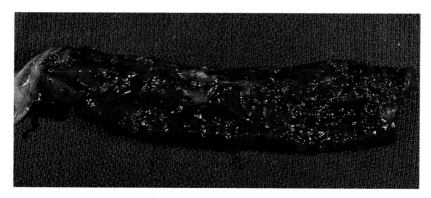

Figure 5-4. On the right side of the placenta slice in the central portion of the villous tissue is a rounded depression. This is a site of maternal blood injection into the intervillous space, a normal finding. The placenta is also very deep red, which is usually due to congestion of fetal villous vessels with blood. While this could reflect fetal circulatory abnormalities, it is commonly caused by early cord clamping. Dark placentas also occur in some cases of maternal diabetes and with certain microscopic villous vascular abnormalities (e.g., chorangiosis). Such villous tissue may feel unusually soft, particularly in the abnormal deep red placentas.

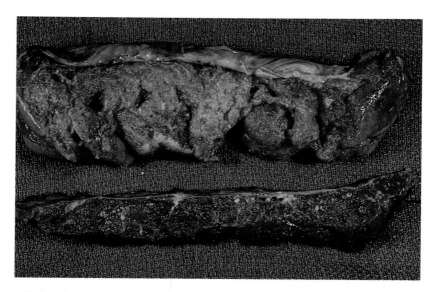

Figure 5-5. A transverse slice of an hydropic placenta (*top*) is compared with a normal term placenta. Extreme pallor is usually present in hydropic placentas, due to factors including fetal anemia, villous edema, and inappropriately immature villous histology. Such placentas are large and thick with coarse villous structure. Hydrops in this case was due to chromosomal aneuploidy.

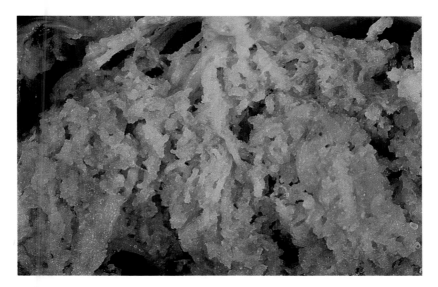

Figure 5-6. A close view of a fixed piece of an hydropic placenta better shows the coarse villous structure. Such placentas may be extremely friable. The pallor here is marked. Placentas will also appear pale if they have lost most of their fetal blood either before or after delivery (draining the cord, villous disruption). In contrast to hydrops, the gross villous size is normal.

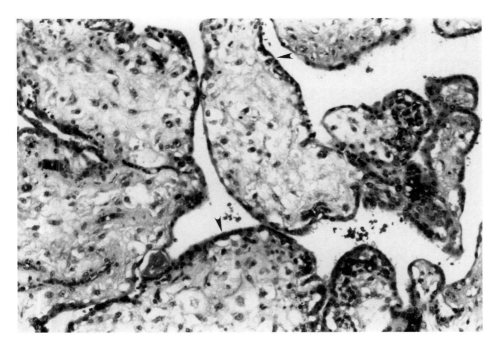

Figure 5-7. Microscopically, these hydropic villi show unusually large size for this near full-term gestation (compare with Figure 2-11, same magnification). The stroma is abundant and edematous. The covering trophoblastic layer shows few syncytial knots, and cytotrophoblasts are easily identified (*arrowheads*), features of abnormal immaturity. There are no specific diagnostic features. The infant showed premature closure of the ductus arteriosus.

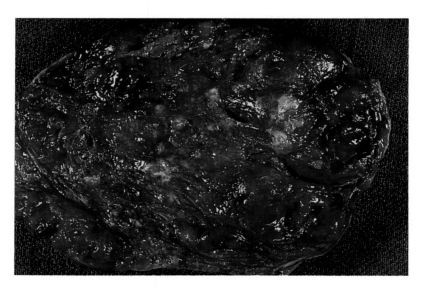

Figure 5-8. The maternal surface of this 30 week placenta reveals many infarcts, yellow polygonal areas which feel quite firm. The villous tissue appears dark and mature (see Figure 5-16). Such placentas are often quite small. Areas of retroplacental blood clot are also identifiable at 2, 4, and 11 o'clock. Placentas with substantial infarction frequently show premature separation, both processes reflecting maternal vascular disease.

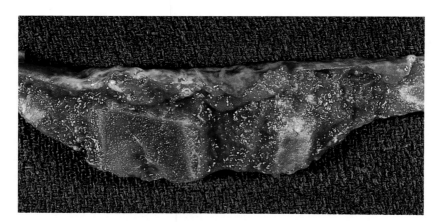

Figure 5-9. Cross section of a multiply infarcted placenta highlights two central lesions. Infarcts are usually square and based on the maternal surface. There is a spared region under the fetal surface due to cross-circulation between districts. Villous collapse leads to the granular appearance, while color reflects the age of the lesion and degeneration of blood. The dark red lesion is relatively recent. The smaller, paler one has been present longer. Portions of other older lesions are seen at the edges. The actual time course of these changes is unknown.

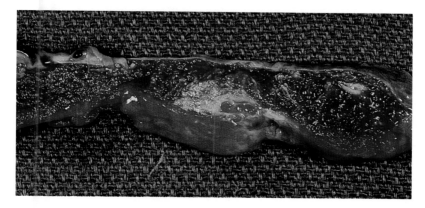

Figure 5-10. This is an old white central infarct. Cystic change may occur and is present here near the base. Infarcts can also show hemorrhagic areas.

Later there is loss of nuclear staining, first of the trophoblast and finally of the entire villus. Fibrin deposits in the intervillous space, but true organization never occurs (Figure 5-14). Maternal vascular lesions can be seen histologically in the basal decidua of some placentas with infarcts (Figure 5-15). Associated ischemic villous pathology is also frequent (Figure 5-16). Vascular disease in the placenta is an important association with growth retardation and preterm delivery.

RETROPLACENTAL HEMORRHAGE

Blood clots on the maternal surface of the placenta are caused by bleeding from decidual vessels in areas of premature placental separation (Figure

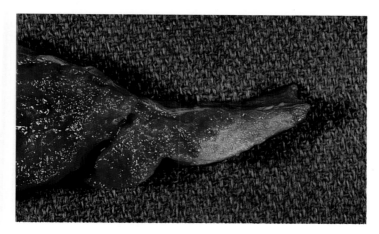

Figure 5-11. Old marginal infarcts are very common, reflecting the poor perfusion near the edge of the placenta. Small lesions such as this are of little significance. Similar infarction often occurs in succenturiate lobes.

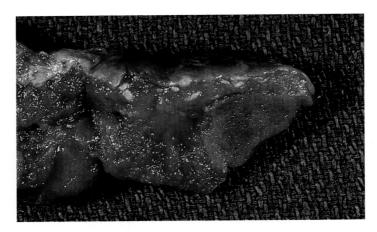

Figure 5-12. A fresh marginal infarct can just be distinguished from the denser nature of the parenchyma of this triangular lesion. Such very recent infarcts are often better palpated than seen.

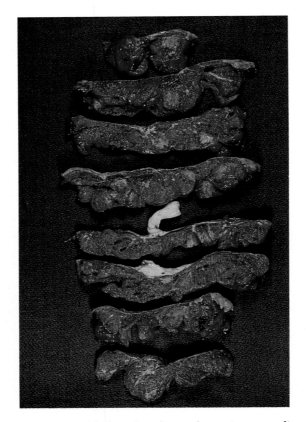

Figure 5-13. The extent of infarction in a placenta can often be better defined if serial slabs are observed simultaneously. Rough quantitation of the percentage of the placenta involved can then be done. Fetal problems such as growth retardation are often present with 15% or more infarction.

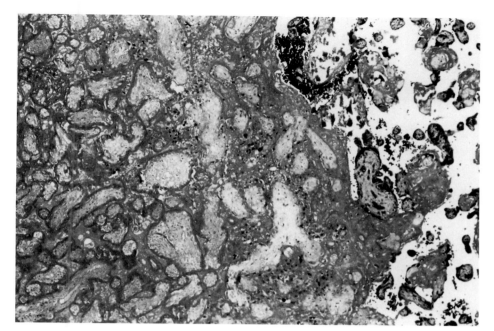

Figure 5-14. Histology of an old infarct reveals ghost outlines of villi enmeshed in fibrin. Nuclear staining has been lost in all the trophoblast and most of the remainder of the villi. Intact villi are present adjacent to the infarct on the right.

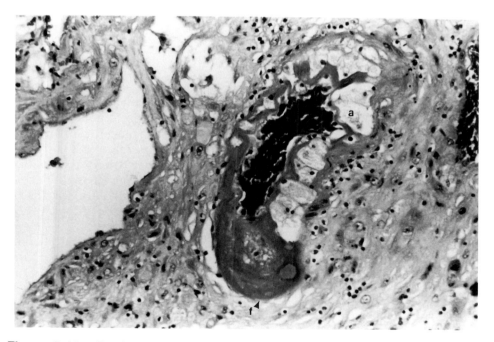

Figure 5-15. Decidual vessels at the base or in the attached decidua may show vascular lesions characteristic of maternal hypertensive disease. This vessel from a severe preeclamptic shows atherosis, a vasculopathy characterized by dense fibrin deposition (f) and lipid-filled atherotic cells (a).

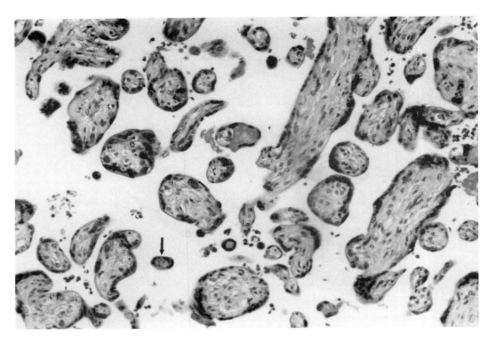

Figure 5-16. Villous structure is often altered in noninfarcted areas of placentas associated with maternal vascular disease. The villi are smaller than expected for gestation with dark smudgy syncytial knots, a change sometimes called "accelerated maturation." Extremely small villi may be present (*arrow*).

5-17), and may relate to significant maternal or fetal disease. Trauma, hypertensive disorders, chorioamnionitis, smoking, and possibly cocaine use have been associated with retroplacental hemorrhage. It is preferable to use descriptive terms for this process rather than "abruptio placenta," a clinical expression implying pain and bleeding. Although some retroplacental hemorrhages correspond to clinical abruptio placenta, many grossly identified hematomas are unsuspected. Also, very recent and at times massive placental separation often has little, if any, gross or histologic change, appearing to be a normally separated placenta. Excessive blood clot received with such a specimen may suggest this.

The gross morphology of retroplacental hemorrhage depends on the duration and degree of blood trapping. When bleeding is contained behind the placenta, the villous tissue becomes compressed by clot (Figure 5-18). If the pregnancy continues, this region infarcts because its blood supply has been lost. Lesions may be subtle on the maternal surface and better seen on cross section (Figure 5-19). Over time the blood breaks down and the infarcts age (Figures 5-20 and 5-21). The exact time course for these placental changes to occur is unknown. When the blood has a means of egress, villous tissue may not be compressed (Figure 5-22). The blood comprising the clots is largely maternal, frequently with some fetal bleeding.

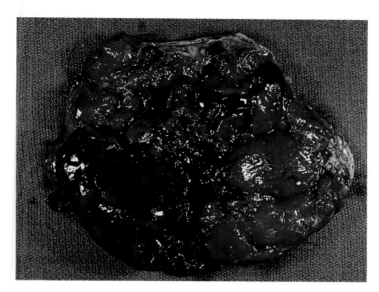

Figure 5-17. Inspection of the uncut maternal surface is the primary means of recognizing retroplacental hemorrhages. This large fresh raised hematoma covers about 25% of the maternal surface and is readily identified. Usually, genuine fresh retroplacental hemorrhage is at least slightly adherent to the maternal surface, as compared with soft postpartum clot. It is also often somewhat granular.

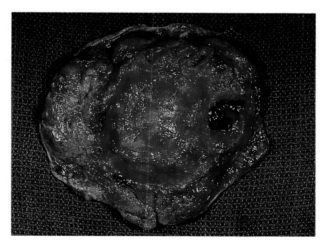

Figure 5-18. In large retroplacental hemorrhages, the clot may become separated from the placenta. A depressed cavity on the maternal surface remains into which the loose clot will often conform. This placenta was associated with a recent intrauterine fetal demise. The large area of placental separation is marked only by the depressed placental tissue.

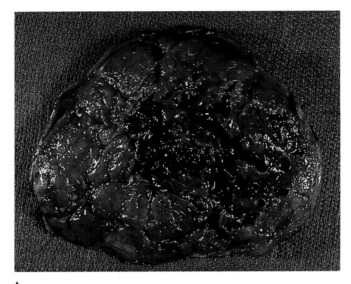

A

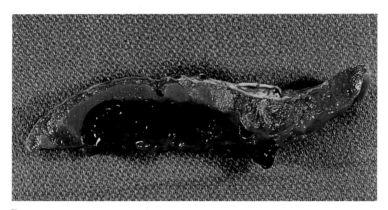

B

Figure 5-19. (a) This retroplacental hemorrhage is subtle. It involves the central portion of the placenta, but is not raised above the surface. Only careful inspection distinguishes it from the surrounding villous tissue. Identification of small lesions of this type requires thorough thoughtful examination. (b) Cross section of the same placenta clearly reveals the nature of the process. Trapping of maternal blood led to the large retroplacental clot which compressed the villous tissue. The villi above the blood are solid and pale, having infarcted from the lack of maternal blood supply. The blood does not show significant degeneration.

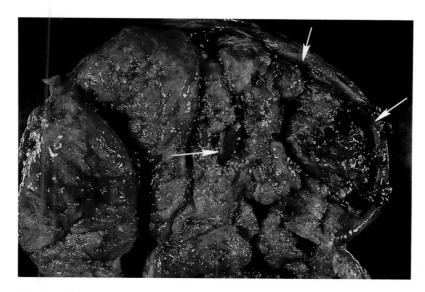

Figure 5-20. Older retroplacental hemorrhages may be very hard to distinguish. Red-tan areas on the maternal surface are regions of old blood clot (*arrows*). The flat yellow areas are attached maternal decidua, a common finding.

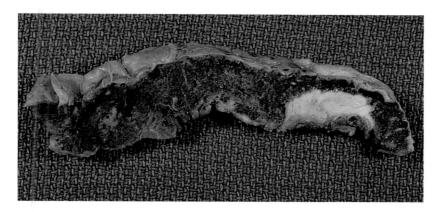

Figure 5-21. Careful examination of the maternal surface of all infarcts is important. This cross section of a fixed placenta shows what appears to be an old infarct. Closer examination of the maternal surface, however, reveals a small amount of red-tan clot, indicating that the lesion is an old retroplacental hemorrhage rather than a simple infarct.

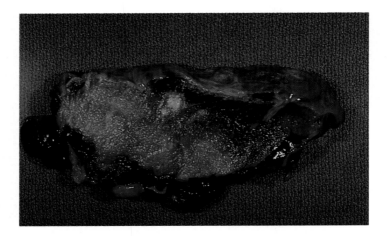

Figure 5-22. In this cross section of another type of retroplacental hemorrhage, there is clot on the surface without villous compression. This occurs if blood has a means of egress. Again there is pallor and infarction of the villous tissue adjacent to the clot. This separation involved nearly the entire placenta and led to fetal demise. A small old yellow infarct near the fetal surface suggests preexisting vascular disease.

Retroplacental hematomas occur both centrally and at the margin of the placenta and overlap villous tissue. True marginal hemorrhage is peripheral, with the aggregate of blood extending onto the membranes (Figures 5-23 and 5-24). It is a fundamentally different process, related to marginal sinus hemorrhage.

INTERVILLOUS THROMBI

Intervillous thrombi occur in the intervillous space in central or basal areas. The earliest thrombi are fresh red clots. These progress through laminated thrombi to old white lesions (Figures 5-25, 5-26, and 5-27). No true organization occurs. Intervillous thrombi contain both fetal and maternal red blood cells. They are seen more frequently in hydrops and other conditions with large friable placentas. The etiology of these lesions is not clear, but may relate to coagulation at sites of villous damage and fetal bleeding.

ATROPHY

Villous atrophy implies interruption of the fetal blood supply. After fetal demise, the entire placenta atrophies if delivery does not occur. It does not

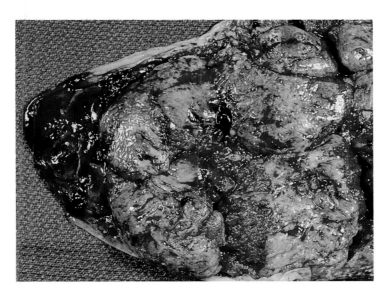

Figure 5-23.   Marginal hemorrhage is present in this preterm placenta. It extends onto the membranes and not the villous tissue. The brown color of the blood indicates it is breaking down. These hemorrhages come from marginal sinus bleeding and not placental separation. They are usually not a problem for the mother or fetus. Note the pale attached decidua on the maternal surface.

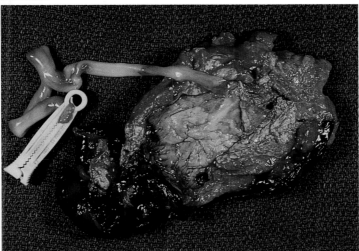

Figure 5-24.   This large marginal hemorrhage occurred in an immature placenta. The fetal surface is yellow-green from severe chorioamnionitis. Many severely infected pregnancies deliver prematurely. The placentas often show severe hemorrhage at the margin, possibly from necrosis of the infected decidua. This is likely a peripartum event, and not the cause of early delivery. The described association of "abruption" with chorioamnionitis is partially due to cases such as this.

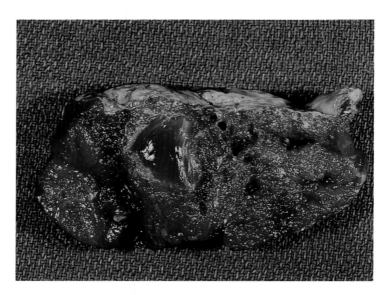

Figure 5-25. Intervillous thrombi will be palpable as firm lesions in the placental tissue. They are shinier and more homogenous in texture than infarcts. Thrombi are usually located in the midportion of the placenta. Color is dependent on age, similar to infarcts. There is some breakdown of blood apparent in this example.

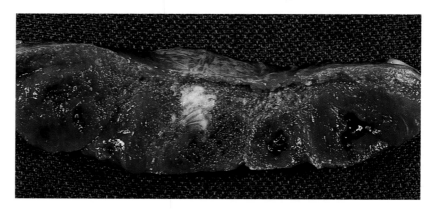

Figure 5-26. This is an older thrombus. Lines of Zahn can be seen in the lower thrombotic portion. The upper section has the granular nature of infarct. Infarction is often noted adjacent to thrombi as the lesions apparently interfere with local villous blood supply. Such associated infarction does not imply maternal vascular disease. Note also the three holes in the villous tissue which are sites of injection of maternal blood.

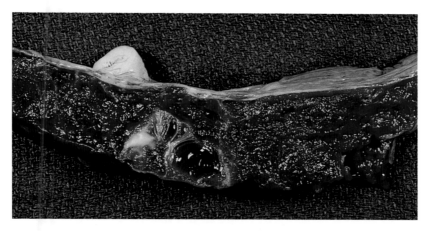

Figure 5-27. This basal intervillous thrombus appears to have several components of different ages. The deep red portion is fresh while the layered material is older. Thrombi occur at the base of the placenta, and should not be confused with retroplacental hemorrhage.

infarct since maternal perfusion continues. Occlusion of only part of the fetal circulation, as with thrombosis, will lead to zones of atrophy, often recognizable grossly (Figures 5-28 and 5-29). Such changes may reflect more diffuse fetal thrombotic processes *in utero,* with the potential for vascular disruptive lesions. Early microscopic change in villi includes vascular breakdown ("hemorrhagic endovasculitis") progressing to complete stromal fibrosis (Figure 5-30). These histologic changes take days to weeks to develop.

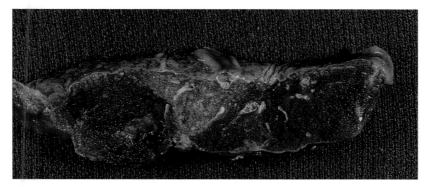

Figure 5-28. The triangular pale region in this placenta is villous atrophy, associated with a large thrombus in a fetal surface vessel. The pale color comes from a lack of fetal blood within the affected villi (same placenta as Figure 4-29).

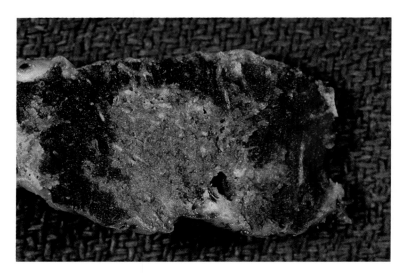

Figure 5-29. Fixed placenta with an irregular pale area of atrophy. No gross thrombosis was noted, which is quite common. There may, however, be fetal vascular changes histologically.

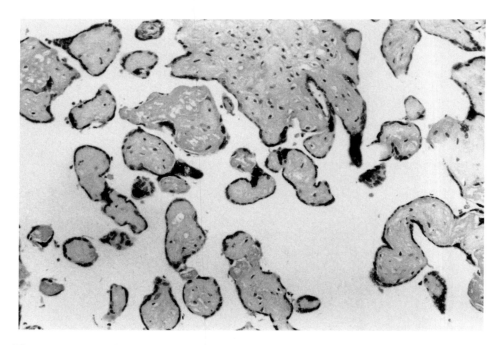

Figure 5-30. Histology of atrophic villi reveals a fibrotic stroma without blood vessels. The trophoblast on the surface is viable since it is still perfused by maternal blood. Change of this degree likely takes more than a week to evolve.

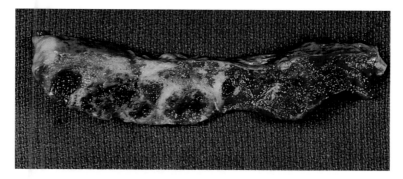

Figure 5-31. The white material deposited in this term placenta is fibrin. Such localized fibrin is common in later gestation. It is deposited in the intervillous space around villi in a lacelike fashion, and usually is quite hard and shiny. Although the entrapped villi eventually die, this process is not generally thought to be related to fetal or maternal disease, apparently originating from turbulence in the maternal circulation. At times, relatively large regions are involved, as shown here. The process, however, is still localized.

FIBRIN DEPOSITION

Some localized areas of perivillous fibrin deposition are seen in virtually all mature placentas (Figure 5-31). Occasionally such deposition is excessive, diffusely involving half or more of the villous tissue (Figure 5-32). This degree is abnormal, and associated with preterm delivery, growth retardation, and death. "Maternal floor infarction" is a related lesion (Figures 5-33 and 5-34). This is not true infarction, consisting of a layer of bland fibrin deposition around basal villi. It has similar associations to diffuse fibrin deposition and can be recurrent. The etiology of maternal floor infarction is unknown, but may be immunologic. Placentas with excess fibrin, both normal and pathologic, often show surface and septal cysts due to the trophoblastic proliferation which occurs in areas of fibrin. The cysts form within trophoblast (Figure 5-35).

CHORANGIOMAS

Chorangiomas are hemangiomas of the placenta and occur in about 1% of pregnancies (Figure 5-36a). They are better designated as hamartomas as they are not true tumors. These lesions commonly occur under the chorionic surface (Figure 5-36b) and have a variety of appearances, depending on vessel size, perfusion, and viability (Figures 5-37, 5-38, and 5-39). Chorangiomas are often confused with other gross lesions (Figure 5-40).

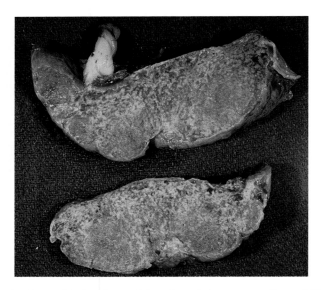

Figure 5-32. Diffuse fibrin deposition involving more than 50% of the placenta is considered abnormal, and is associated with prematurity, fetal growth retardation, and death. The etiology is unknown. This thick, immature, very pale placenta shows a diffuse network of fibrin, and was associated with intrauterine demise at 25 weeks of a poorly grown infant. Such placentas are usually quite firm.

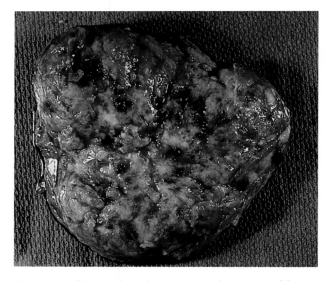

Figure 5-33. Maternal floor of an immature placenta with excess fibrin deposition shows firm yellow plaques. Such an appearance is suggestive of maternal floor infarction, which is better visualized on cut sections.

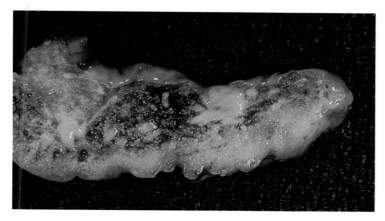

Figure 5-34. In "maternal floor infarction" there is a layer of fibrin deposited at the base for 3–4 mm. Basal villi are entrapped and die, but it is not true infarction. Diffuse intervillous fibrin is often present. This recurring lesion is associated with growth retardation and death. The placenta shown is from a 25 week stillborn, however infants may be liveborn.

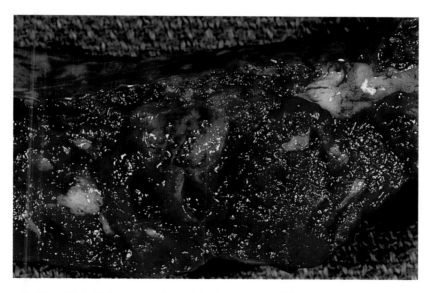

Figure 5-35. This thin-walled cyst is located within a septum of a term placenta. Such cysts also occur on the surface (Figure 4-17). They develop in the presence of abundant fibrin deposition, but do not appear to be associated intrinsically with any pathology.

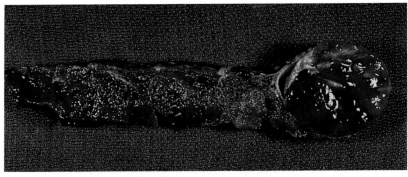

A

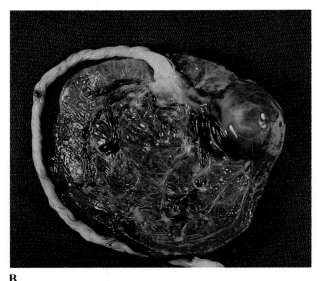

B

Figure 5-36. (a) The red, round solid lesion at the right side of this term placental section is a chorangioma or hemangioma of the placenta. These are usually nodular, fleshy lesions. (b) Surface view of the placenta prior to cutting shows that the chorangioma originally appeared as a raised, sub-chorionic nodule. This is a common location and causes confusion on ultrasound with cysts and large, nodular, subchorionic hematomas (Figures 4-3 and 4-18).

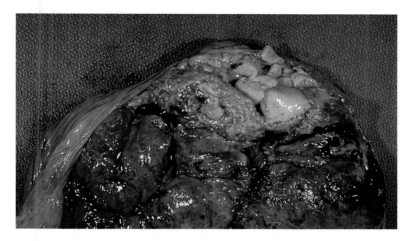

Figure 5-37. Another chorangioma in a preterm placenta is much paler and irregularly lobulated. The size of the vessels, their congestion, and the presence of infarction will determine the color of the mass. Large chorangiomas such as this may be associated with nonimmune hydrops, possibly caused by fetal circulatory overload and shunting. Trapping of platelets and fetal thrombocytopenia may also occur.

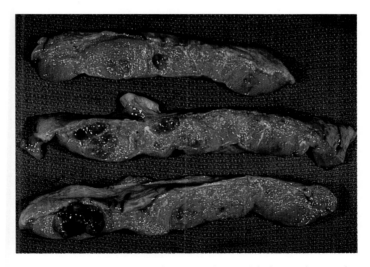

Figure 5-38. Chorangiomas are frequently multiple and may be pedunculated, as shown by the multiple berry-like lesions here.

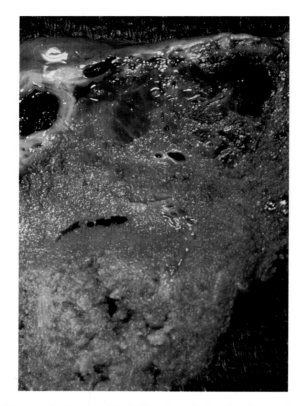

Figure 5-39. The gelatinous ill-defined subchorionic region in this fixed placenta was histologically a chorangioma.

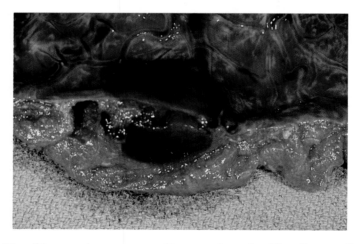

Figure 5-40. Chorangiomas are often confused with other pathologic lesions. This thrombus-like mass was actually a chorangioma. Infarction in the lesion may give this appearance.

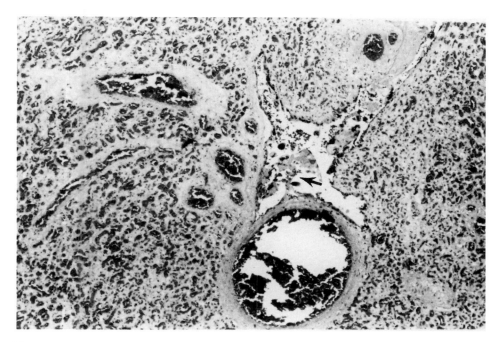

Figure 5-41. Microscopic view of a chorangioma reveals numerous small and a few larger blood vessels in lobulated areas resembling large villi. The vessels are congested. The surface of the chorangiomatous nodules is covered by trophoblast which, as usual, is somewhat hyperplastic (*arrow*).

Histology is that of a typical hemangioma, usually with small or medium sized vessels (Figure 5-41). Large chorangiomas may lead to fetal hydrops and platelet trapping. Rarely the infants have other hemangiomas.

INFLAMMATORY VILLOUS LESIONS

Infections reaching the infant from the mother's bloodstream will traverse the villi. Examples of this include rubella, cytomegalovirus, and syphilis. Usually no specific infectious gross lesions are identifiable, although the placenta may be hydropic or unusually firm and fibrotic. *Listeria monocytogenes,* however, also infects by the hematogenous route and typically causes grossly visible necrotizing abscesses (Figure 5-42). Rarely other infectious lesions are identified in the villous tissue (Figure 5-43). Much of the villous inflammatory disease identified histologically is nonspecific villitis, most likely a lesion of immunologic rather than infectious origin (Figure 5-44).

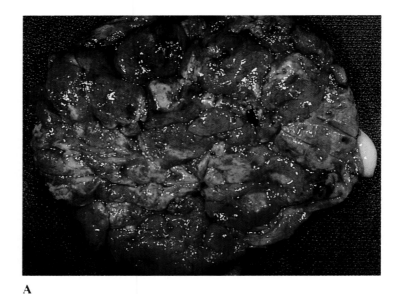

A

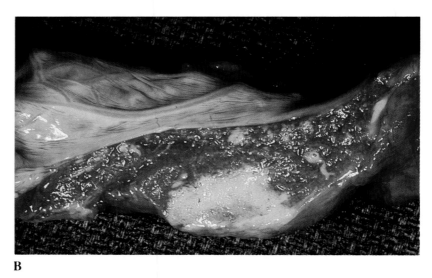

B

Figure 5-42. (a) The maternal surface of a 26 week placenta infected with listeria shows numerous yellow-white lesions, reminiscent of infarcts. The villous tissue, however, appear pale and immature, unusual when there is early severe vascular disease. This suggests a different process. The areas are actually abscesses. (b) Cross section of one abscess also suggests infarction. Smaller lesions dispersed diffusely in the villi also occur (upper right). Listeria is usually associated with severe chorioamnionitis, and the fetal surface here is opaque.

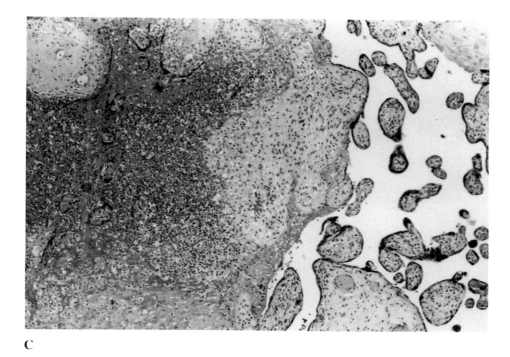

C

Figure 5-42. (c) Microscopy of these lesions shows extensive acute inflammation. There is necrosis and some villous ghosts, contributing to the infarctive appearance.

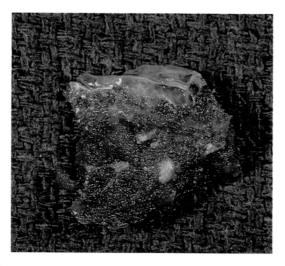

Figure 5-43. Cross-sections of a placenta occasionally reveal round, soft yellow lesions only a few millimeters wide. Such areas may be small abscesses. Listeria or other organisms may be involved. The lesion depicted was histologically granulomatous and occurred in a woman with AIDS and disseminated tuberculosis. Acid-fast bacteria were abundant.

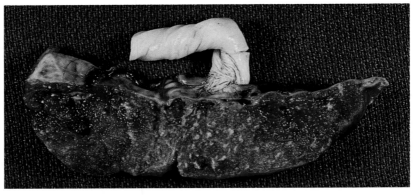

A

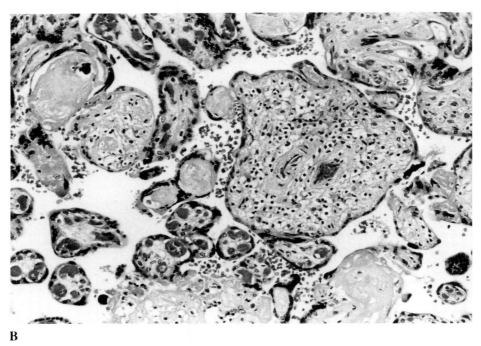

B

Figure 5-44. (a) Nonspecific villous inflammation (villitis of unknown etiology) is not usually identifiable grossly. Occasionally placentas with severe disease will have visible abnormalities. These resemble fibrin deposition and/ or atrophy, often with a yellow color and more granular nature as shown here. On histology this placenta showed nonspecific inflammatory changes involving half the villi. (b) Histology of nonspecific villitis shows villi enlarged with inflammatory cells (lymphocytes) admixed with normal villi. The fetal vasculature is obliterated in areas, which leads to the atrophic appearance. Fibrin deposition and villous agglutination may also be features. Villitis is associated with a variable degree of growth retardation and can be recurrent.

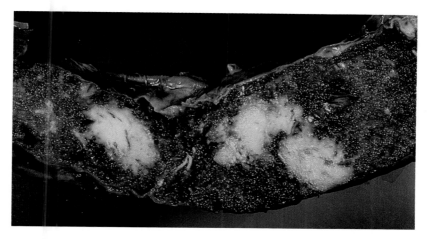

Figure 5-45. While careful examination of gross placental lesions is usually diagnostic, some will remain enigmas until microscopy is done. This fixed placenta shows numerous round white lesions which are not typical of infarct, thrombus, chorangioma, atrophy, or fibrin deposition. Histology revealed them to be infarcts, in a placenta with other changes of maternal vascular disease.

HISTOLOGIC STUDY

While inspection will definitively identify the majority of gross villous lesions, occasional cases are unclear until microscopy has been performed (Figures 5-40 and 5-45). Histologic confirmation of those gross processes likely to be associated with fetal or maternal disease should also be done. Isolated infarcts or thrombi do not require further study, particularly in term placentas.

6
MULTIPLE GESTATIONS

One in 100 births is a multiple gestation, making the examination of these placentas one of the most important aspects of placental pathology. Twins account for a disproportionate percentage of perinatal morbidity and mortality, with significantly higher rates than singletons. Placentas of multiple gestations demonstrate all the abnormalities seen in singletons, as well as their own special pathology. This is even truer in higher multiple births, which are becoming more common with assisted reproductive techniques. While most of the following discussion relates to twins, the same principles are used when evaluating triplet and quadruplet placentas. Special twin report forms are useful (Appendix A-3).

CHORIONICITY

Determination of the chorionicity of a twin placenta is the most important step in examination (Figure 6-1). "Dichorionic" means two placentas have formed, while "monochorionic" indicates a single shared placenta. Any gestation arising from two separate fertilized eggs will be dichorionic, as each conception has its own placenta. The placentas may be totally separate, however, limitations of space in the uterus frequently lead to fusion and a single disk.

Monochorionic placentas occur only in monozygotic or "identical" twins. The fertilized egg splits early in gestation and each portion continues to develop separately. Splits occurring before 3 days of development lead to gestations with totally separate placentas, as all the cells of the conceptus are undifferentiated. At about 3 days some cells become developmentally committed as trophoblast and can no longer split. This leads to two separate embryos and amnions developing within a single chorion. Later splits are unusual and lead to twins in a single amniotic sac (monoamnionic) and finally conjoined twins. Two-thirds of monozygotic twins are monochorionic, and the remainder dichorionic. The like-sexed monozygotic dichorionic

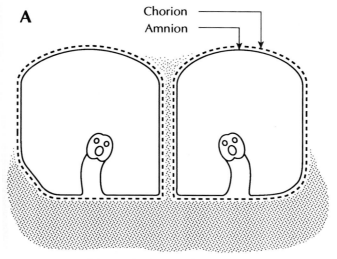

Diamniotic Dichorionic
(fused)

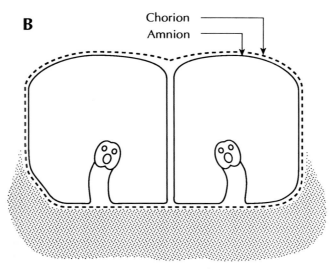

Diamniotic Monochorionic

Figure 6-1. Diagrammatic views of the types of fused twin placentas with two amniotic sacs. (a) The dichorionic placenta has two sacs each enclosed by amnion and chorion. There is chorionic tissue (stipples) in the dividing membranes, forming a ridge on the surface. (b) The monochorionic placenta shows no chorionic material in the dividing membranes, the chorion forming a continuous plate on the surface of the placenta. The dividing membranes consist of only two amnions.

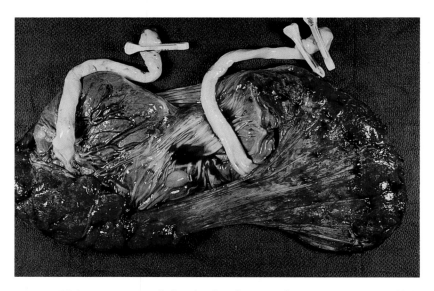

Figure 6-2. This near term dichorionic placenta has two separate disks connected by membranes. A draped piece of thick, dividing membrane can be seen between the cords. Note the fresh meconium on the dividing membranes on the side of B (two clamps).

twins cannot be differentiated from the like-sexed dizygotic dichorionic twins by placental exam. Only genetic testing will definitively distinguish them. In the United States about 80% of like-sexed dichorionic twins are dizygotic, based on the incidence of twin types. The incidence of monozygotic twins is constant throughout the world (1/300 births). The incidence of dizygotic twins is quite variable. These twins may be familial.

EXAMINATION OF TWIN PLACENTAS

Separate twin placentas, which are always dichorionic, are examined as one would singleton placentas. In fused placentas, gross determination of the chorionicity is quite simple. The dividing membranes between the twins are evaluated for thickness and opacity. Dichorionic membranes are relatively thick and opaque (Figure 6-2), and there is a ridge where the dividing membranes meet the placenta (Figure 6-3). If one tries to completely remove dichorionic dividing membranes by separating the layers, the placental surface will be disrupted. In contrast, the nearly transparent membranes of monochorionic placentas show no ridge and are easily separated leaving a continuous monochorionic plate (Figures 6-4 and 6-5).

Chorionicity can be histologically confirmed in two ways. "T" sections include dividing membranes and a point where they reach the placental

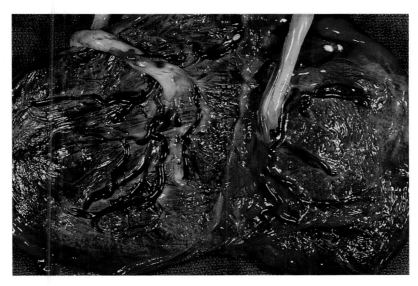

Figure 6-3. The dividing membranes have been largely removed on this placenta with a fused disk. Note the ridge of chorionic tissue between the cords where the membranes had met the surface. This is diagnostic of a dichorionic placenta. The vessels of each side do not connect.

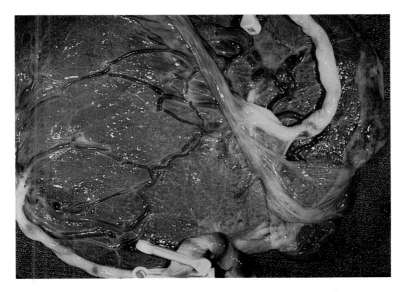

Figure 6-4. The extremely thin and delicate dividing membranes are folded on the surface of this monochorionic placenta. Note how little substance they have. Vessels dispersing from the cords can be seen to connect at the left side of the placental surface. Only monochorionic placentas have vascular anastomoses. The cord on the right shows an amniotic web.

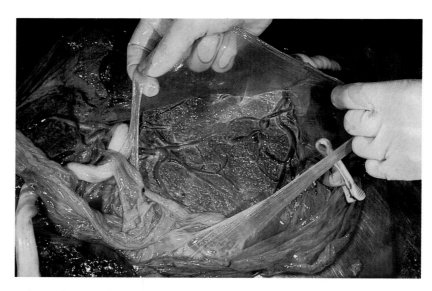

Figure 6-5. The dividing membranes of a monochorionic placenta can be readily separated, leaving a smooth continuous chorionic surface between the two cord insertions. The vascular anastomoses are now more easily seen.

surface. While such sections are readily made on fixed dichorionic placentas, with monochorionic ones the amnions often separate. It is generally easier to make a roll of the dividing membranes similar to what is done with the peripheral membranes (Figure 6-6). The dividing membrane is composed of 3–4 layers in dichorionic twins, and only two layers in monochorionic placentas (Figure 6-7).

Monochorionic placentas virtually always show one or more vascular anastomoses (Figure 6-8). These vascular anastomoses lead to the specific problems of monozygotic twins, and it is important to document them. Diagrams are useful in complicated cases. Arteries always pass over veins. By just visually following large superficial vessels one will identify most of the vascular connections between the two sides. A small syringe can be used to inject vessels, entering proximal to the presumed point of anastomosis and manually occluding backflow. The water, milk, air, or dye will be seen crossing to the other side. Small deep anastomoses are difficult to identify, and injection may not be successful due to disruption or incomplete filling.

Once chorionicity and vessels are examined, the usual evaluation of the cord, membranes, and villous tissue is done in both mono and dichorionic placentas. The entire placenta is weighed and measured after making membrane rolls and removing the cords and extra membranes. The placenta is then divided along the approximate vascular plane by cutting in monochorionic placentas or by traction and separation in dichorionic ones. Each portion is weighed. Differences between the twins such as villous color should be noted. Tissue from each is placed in its own container. Hopefully the

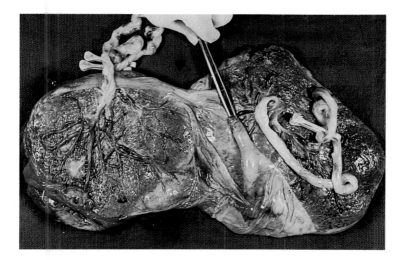

Figure 6-6. Documentation of chorionicity is most easily done with a roll of the dividing membranes made in the same manner as a peripheral membrane roll. The placenta shown is dichorionic with two separate disks. Such placentas often deliver completely separate, without fused dividing membranes to sample.

cords have been labeled. If not, they should be arbitrarily designated and the materials kept separate. The usual routine placenta blocks are submitted using villous tissue clearly from the region of each twin. Sections of the junctional zone may highlight differences in villous structure.

PROBLEMS UNIQUE TO MONOCHORIONIC TWINS

The vascular anastomoses virtually always present in monochorionic placentas cause special problems. Unbalanced cross-circulation can lead to the transfusion syndrome. In chronic cases the classic presentation is an anemic, growth-retarded donor twin with oligohydramnios and a larger, plethoric recipient with polyhydramnios. Hydrops may occur in either infant. The donor has a pale placenta from anemia (Figure 6-9). The recipient's placenta is deep red and congested. There may be microscopic differences in villous structure and maturation, which are usually subtle, even in clearcut chronic transfusions. Acute transfusion syndromes also occur. One fetus can bleed through the anastomoses into the placenta of the other when pressures drop after the first is delivered. At times this can reverse the gross appearance of a chronic transfusion (Figure 6-10). Careful evaluation and documentation of the placental anastomoses is particularly important in such cases.

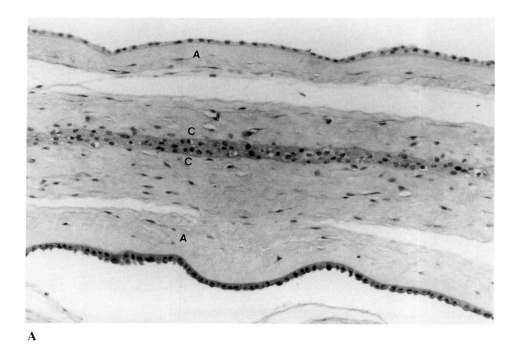

A

B

Figure 6-7. (a) Microscopic view of dividing membranes in a roll from a dichorionic twin gestation shows that they are composed of amnion from each twin containing epithelial cells and attached connective tissue (A) and chorion from each in which the two chorionic layers may fuse (C). Any chorionic tissue in the dividing membranes indicates a dichorionic placenta. (b) Dividing membranes of a monochorionic gestation only shows two layers of amnion (A).

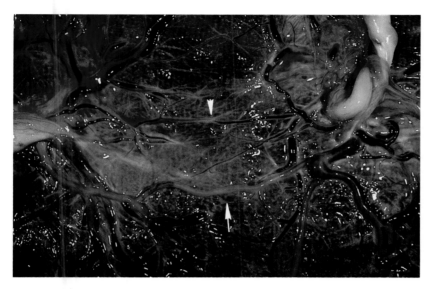

Figure 6-8. Vascular anastomoses in a monochorionic placenta are shown after removal of the amnion. The lower anastomosis (*arrow*) shows large arteries from each cord fusing in the center. The vessels, clear from injected water, are recognized as arteries because they pass over other vessels. Injection is usually not necessary to identify such large connections. Above this (*arrow head*) is an area suggestive of a deep artery-vein connection. Arteries and veins usually run together as pairs. Here, an artery from the left cord ends without a parallel returning vessel. A similar vein from the right ends just adjacent to it. While such anastomoses are important and most implicated in transfusion syndrome, they are difficult to inject because of pressure or disruption in the circuit. Recognition of their usual gross morphology is thus important.

Very premature delivery is common in severe transfusion syndromes, often occurring in the second trimester. If one twin dies, the situation may resolve when cross-circulation ceases (Figure 6-11). Vascular disruptive abnormalities such as gut atresia and porencephalic cysts occur in about 20% of the surviving twins. It is believed that circulatory changes similar to those in acute transfusion syndrome occur around the time of death and cause damage at that time. The incidence of disruptions in the survivor does not increase with long duration of the pregnancy after the demise. The possibility of similar damage to the surviving twin has tempered enthusiasm for therapeutic reduction in cases of transfusion syndrome. Techniques for actual obliteration of the problematic anastomoses are in development.

A special set of anastomoses permits the development of acardiac twins (Figure 6-12). Such fetuses are passively perfused by their co-twin and lack cardiac development from the circulatory reversal. External and internal development is strikingly abnormal.

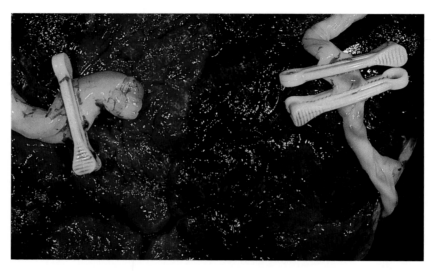

Figure 6-9. The maternal surface of this monochorionic placenta shows changes that may be present with transfusion syndrome. There is a difference in color between the two sides. The paler region was associated with the anemic donor twin.

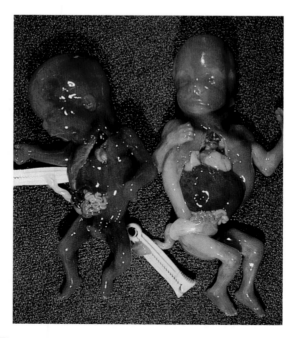

Figure 6-10. These two 17 week fetuses show evidence of both acute and chronic transfusion syndrome. The larger fetus has a hypertrophied heart, evidence of recipient status in chronic transfusion syndrome. It is, however, quite pale, having acutely bled most of its blood volume into the smaller twin (chronic donor, acute recipient).

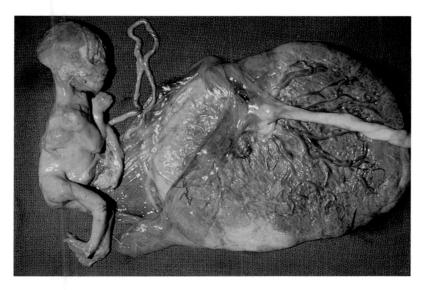

Figure 6-11. Death of one twin at 19 weeks led to the formation of a fetus papyraceous. Morphology was adequately preserved to permit the histologic confirmation of the dividing membranes as monochorionic. While the etiology of the death of the infant is not fully determinable at this time, transfusion syndrome is most likely. The surviving twin was at increased risk for vascular disruptive anomalies, but was uninvolved. The pregnancy went to term.

A small portion of monochorionic twin placentas entail relatively late splits in the conceptus. Placentas with a single, shared amniotic sac are prone to cord entanglement with high morbidity and mortality (Figures 6-13 and 6-14).

ABNORMALITIES FOUND IN ALL TWIN PLACENTAS

Differences between twins are common in both mono and dichorionic placentas, and are frequently not due to the special aspects of monochorionic twins. Placental anomalies account for some of the perinatal problems observed in multiple gestations. Some are due to limitations of space in the uterus. Abnormal cord insertions are far more common (Figure 6-15). Single umbilical arteries and succenturiate lobes are frequent. Differences in placental size can be associated with growth retardation (Figure 6-16). Other pathologic processes may differentially affect the two placentas. Ascending infection is common (Figure 6-17).

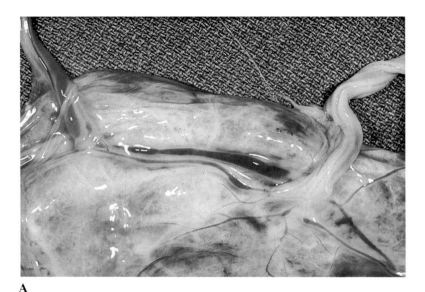

A

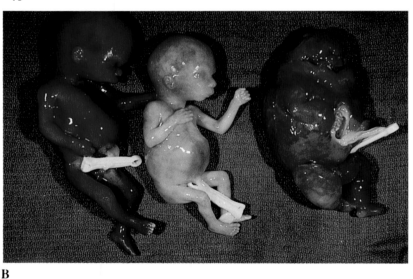

B

Figure 6-12. (a) Single artery-to-artery and vein-to-vein anastomoses near the cords connected two of the fetuses in this set of monochorionic triplets at 19 weeks. Such anastomoses permit circulatory reversal in one of the pair, and the possibility of development of an acardiac twin, which occurred in this case. (b) The deep red edematous acardiac twin is present at the right end. Note the much poorer formation of the upper body, which is typical. In the normally formed fetuses, one is quite pale and the other plethoric. A transfusion syndrome occurred between these two. The donor twin was extremely stressed as it also perfused the acardiac.

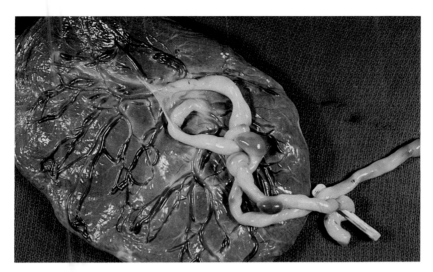

Figure 6-13. This monoamniotic placenta shows a common finding in such twins—entanglement of the cords with knotting. Mortality is said to be 50% in monoamniotic twins, largely from this. Much of this cord-associated mortality occurs early in gestation. Limitation of space in the uterus prevents the necessary tightening after 30 weeks. Vascular anastomoses are usually present in monoamniotic placentas, but tend to be large and transfusion syndrome is uncommon. These infants had no apparent problems and were delivered near term.

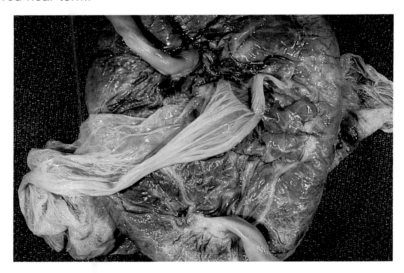

Figure 6-14. The dividing amnion is incomplete in this diamnionic monochorionic placenta, becoming absent near the upper right. This is an amniotic "plica," whose origin is not clear. Split of this conceptus may have occurred slightly earlier here than in a true monoamniotic placenta, with only partial formation of the amnion. It has also been suggested that rupture of the amnion in a diamnionic monochorionic placenta could also lead to this configuration. (Reproduced with permission from Gilbert WM, Davis SE, Kaplan C, et al: Morbidity associated with prenatal disruption of the dividing membrane in twin gestations. *Obstet Gynecol* 78: 623–630, 1991.)

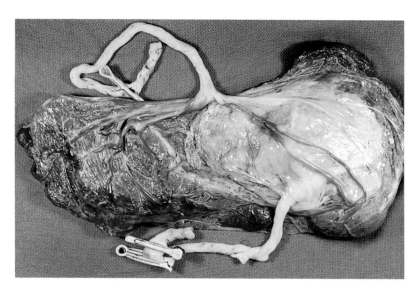

Figure 6-15. Cord abnormalities are very common in multiple gestations, and may lead to asymmetric infants. A complex velamentous cord insertion is present here. The vessels of one cord traverse the dividing membranes to placental tissue on the opposite side of the other disk. Vessels within the dividing membranes only occur in dichorionic placentas. Dividing membrane insertions seem particularly prone to problems including compression and thrombosis.

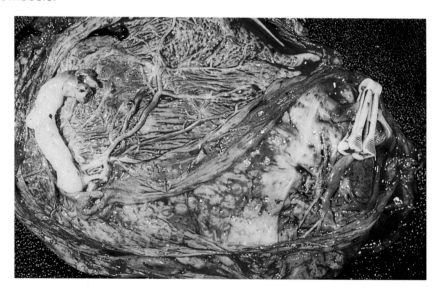

Figure 6-16. This dichorionic placenta (note prominent ridge) shows a marked difference between the sizes of the two placental portions. The smaller placenta was associated with a severely growth-retarded infant. Such discrepancies may be due to unequal placentation caused by problems of space in the uterus, or by a process affecting only one infant (e.g., chromosomal aneuploidy, vascular disease). Similar inequalities occur in monochorionic twins as well.

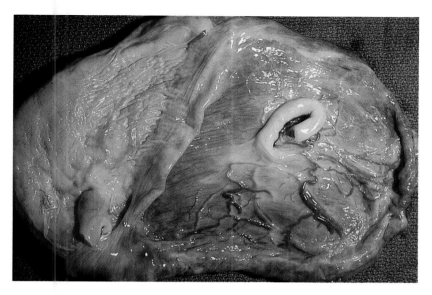

Figure 6-17. Chorioamnionitis is common in multiple gestations. The over-distension of the uterus may increase susceptibility, and infection frequently contributes to early delivery. This very immature dichorionic placenta shows markedly asymmetric chorioamnionitis. The left side, Baby A, shows severe changes with a dense yellow-green surface. The placenta of Baby B is opaci-fied as well, but much less so. Such findings support the ascending theory of origin for chorioamnionitis. The lower infant (A), closer to the cervix, is infected before the upper infant (B), and B will only show ascending infection if it is present in A. This is also true in monochorionic placentas with vascular anastomoses, confirming the nonhematogenous nature of the process.

HIGHER MULTIPLE BIRTHS

The same basic concepts as in twins apply when examining the placentas of higher multiple births. The steps of examining the dividing membranes and making rolls will need to be done several times, once for each pair. The placentas are often quite disrupted (Figure 6-18), and other abnormalities are frequently seen. Many of these deliveries come from assisted fertilization techniques with multiple separate eggs, usually leading to a separate chorion for each infant (Figure 6-19). The incidence of monochorionic gestations is also increased with such manipulations.

In multiple gestations, any fetus which dies is retained as long as the pregnancy continues, leading to a compressed "fetus papyraceous." These occur in both mono and multichorionic gestations, and chorionicity can usu-ally be determined. Although many result from transfusion syndrome, other etiologies include anomalies, cord problems, and reductions of higher multi-ple births (Figures 6-20 and 6-21).

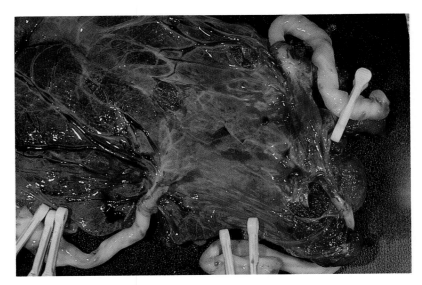

Figure 6-18. Although this triplet placenta is rather disrupted, one can still identify that this is a monochorionic set. There is one continuous chorionic plate with three cords. Even disrupted placentas should be carefully examined as there is often much that can still be identified about their gross morphology.

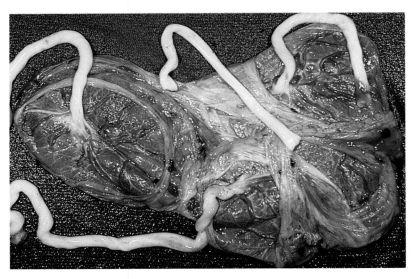

Figure 6-19. This is from a tetrachorionic Pergonal®-induced quadruplet pregnancy. There are four nearly separate placentas of varying sizes. Such placentas can be examined in a manner similar to twin gestations, evaluating each of the dividing membranes and placental regions separately. Unequal placentation is common in higher multiple births.

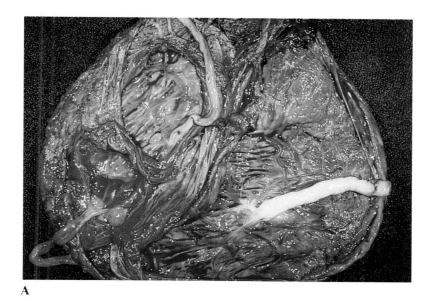

A

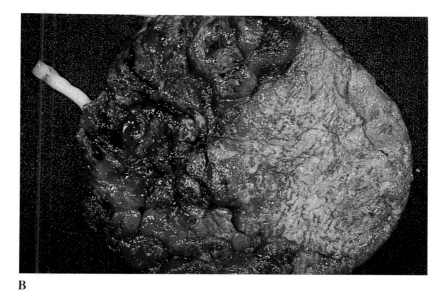

B

Figure 6-20. (a) Two of three fetuses were lost in this naturally occurring set of triplets. The surviving infant was female, while the two demises were male. Detailed examination of the dividing membranes showed them to be monochorionic, and death was probably due to transfusion syndrome. These were biovular triplets, with split of one egg, the most common spontaneous type. (b) Maternal side of this placenta shows the extreme atrophy of the villous tissue belonging to the monochorionic twins (right). Severe changes of fetal demise, including villous atrophy and extensive fibrin deposition, will be present with extremely long retention as occurred here.

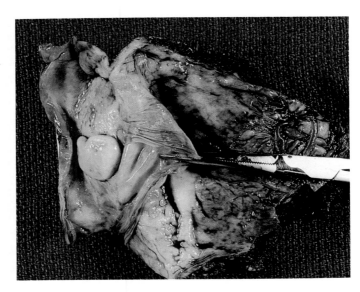

Figure 6-21. With assisted fertilization techniques there is often early loss of one or more conceptions, either spontaneously or through intervention. In this *in vitro* fertilization pregnancy, quintuplets were conceived. Three of the five were reduced at 9 weeks. One fetus papyraceous is shown at the edge of a portion of the fixed placenta. Two others were present. Careful examination is necessary to identify these, as they resemble plaques of fibrin (see Figure 4-34). All five had separate chorions. The remaining dichorionic twins delivered at 35 weeks.

Appendix A-1   GROSS WORKSHEET

                                                       Microscopic

History: Vag/CS   weeks   male/female   grams
meconium/preeclampsia/diabetes

WEIGHT   gm   fixed

CORD   length   cm   cen/ecc/marg/vel   web   cm   true knot/cong
       twist R/L/A   2V   torn cord/vessels   furcate   cm

MEMBRANES   cm   disrupted   absent

    % CIRCUMMARGINATION rim cm   % CIRCUMVALLATION rim cm

SUBCHORIONIC FIBRIN 0/ 1 / 2 / 3   SUBCHORIONIC HEMORRHAGE   % old/recent

OPACITY/GREEN STAINING/HEMOLYSIS/BETADINE/SUBAMNIOTIC HEMORRHAGE
       slight/fresh/thick/edema

DIMENSIONS   ×   ×   cm   BILOBATE   ×   cm   IRREGULAR

SUCCENTURIATE LOBE 1.   ×   ×   cm   2.   ×   ×   cm   atrophic/partial

MATERNAL SURFACE disrupted focal/extensive   CALCIFICATION: 0/ 1 / 2 / 3

THROMBUS   1.   cm   2.   cm   3.   cm   Fresh/Recent/Old

INFARCTS   marginal   1.   cm   2.   cm.   3.   cm

           central   1.   cm   2.   cm.   3.   cm

HEMORR OLD 1. × cm RM/RP mar/ cm   2. × cm RM/RP mar/ cm

           1. × cm RM/RP mar/ cm   2. × cm RM/RP mar/ cm
FRESH/REC

FIBRIN DEPOSITION diffuse   1. x cm   2. × cm

ATROPHY diffuse   1.   ×   cm 2.   ×   cm

pale / deep red / soft / firm

soft clot   grams

<u>Appendix A-2</u>   SINGLETON REPORT FORM

S-   NAME:

History: Vaginal delivery/Cesarean section   weeks;
    gram male/female infant

Received fresh is a   gram placenta with a   cm 3 vessel left twisted
(central/eccentric/marginal/velamentous/furcate) cord with a   cm amniotic
web. Membranes are (incomplete/essentially complete) and ruptured   cm
from the placental margin. Membrane insertion is (at the margin/   % cir-
cummarginate/circumvallate with a rim to   cm).   Subchorionic fibrin is
(minimal/slight/moderate/abundant).   There is (opacity/green coloration/
no unusual coloration) of the fetal surface. The placental disk
is   ×   ×   cm approximate greatest dimensions.   The maternal
surface is (apparently complete/disrupted focally).   There is (no/slight/
moderate/abundant) calcification.   On cut section, color and consistency
are unremarkable. (No) other gross lesions:

> retromembranous/retroplacental hemorrhage
> intervillous thrombus
> succenturiate lobe
> marginal infarct
> central infarct

Soft clot present.

Microscopic performed. Gross only. Tissue blocks available.

DIAGNOSIS:
Placenta, delivery—No pathologic diagnosis (NPD)
    Immaturity
    Ischemic change
    Subchorionic intervillositis/chorionitis/chorioamnionitis
    Retroplacental/marginal hemorrhage
    Intervillous thrombus
    (Marginal) infarct
    Succenturiate lobe

Fetal membranes, delivery—NPD
    Acute inflammation/chorioamnionitis
    Meconium pigmentation
    Retromembranous hemorrhage
    Circumvallate/circummarginate

Umbilical cord, delivery—NPD
    Marginal/velamentous insertion
    Acute phlebitis/vasculitis/funisitis

TWIN REPORT FORM

S-   Name:

Cesarean section/vaginal delivery   weeks

A (1 clamp) male/female   grams   B (2 clamps) male/female   grams

Received fresh is a diamniotic di/monochorionic twin placenta with (separate/fused) disks. Cords are (unlabeled and arbitrarily designated/labeled with 1 and 2 clamps).   Overall the placenta is   grams and   ×   ×   cm. Injection studies are performed revealing   artery-to-artery and artery-to-vein anastomosis from   to   . The placentas are divided along the approximate vascular plane.

I (clamp) is   grams and   ×   ×   cm with a   cm 3 vessel left twisted (central/eccentric/marginal/velamentous) cord. Membranes are (incomplete/ruptured   cm from the margin). There is (opacity/green staining/no unusual color) of the fetal surface. Maternal side is (apparently complete/disrupted focally). (No/slight/moderate) calcification. No other gross lesions.

II (clamps) is   grams and   ×   ×   cm with a   cm 3 vessel left twisted (central/eccentric/marginal/velamentous) cord. Membranes are (incomplete/ruptured   cm. from the margin). There is (opacity/green staining/no unusual color) of the fetal surface. Maternal side is (apparently complete/disrupted focally). (No/slight/moderate) calcification. (No) other gross lesions.

Representative sections including dividing membranes. Microscopic performed.

DIAGNOSIS:

Placenta, delivery—Twins, dichorionic/monochorionic (identical)

          Immaturity

          Subchorionic intervillositis/chorionitis/chorioamnionitis

Fetal membranes, delivery—NPD

          Acute inflammation/chorioamnionitis

Umbilical cord, delivery—NPD

          Marginal/velamentous insertion

          Single artery

          Acute phlebitis/vasculitis/funisitis

Note: Although like-sexed dichorionic twins may be mono or dizygotic, about 80% are dizygotic.

PLACENTAL WEIGHT RATIO

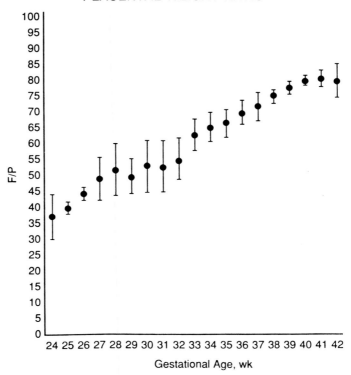

Appendix B-1 Mean fetoplacental weight ratios with 95% confidence limits by gestational age for normally grown infants. (From Molteni RA, Stys SJ, Battaglia FC: Relationship of fetal and placental weight in human beings: Fetal/placental weight ratios at various gestational ages and birth weight distributions. *J Reprod Med* 21 327–334, 1978).

PLACENTAL WEIGHT

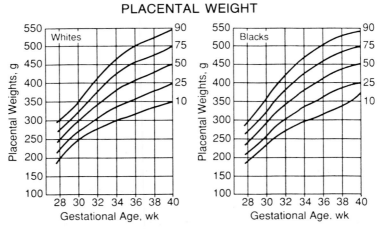

Appendix B-2 Placental growth curves for whites and blacks. (from Naeye RL: Do placental weights have clinical significance? *Hum Pathol* 18:387–391, 1987).

PLACENTAL WEIGHT GRAPH

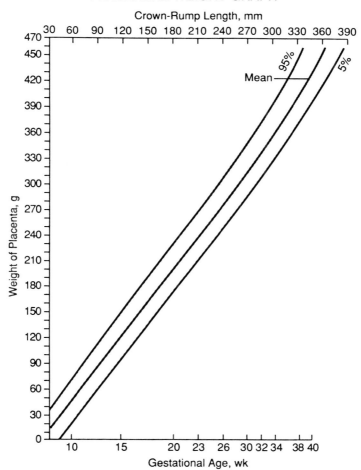

Appendix B-3 Placental weight related to crown-rump length and gestational age. (With permission of Oxford Press from Hall JG, Froster-Iskenius UG, Allanson JE: *Handbook of Normal Physical Measurements.* New York, Oxford University Press, 1989, p. 432).

UMBILICAL CORD LENGTH

Gestational age, wk	n	Umbilical Cord Length, cm
20 to 21	16	32.4 ± 8.6
22 to 23	27	36.4 ± 9.0
24 to 25	38	40.1 ± 10.1
26 to 27	59	42.5 ± 11.3
28 to 29	80	45.0 ± 9.7
30 to 31	113	47.6 ± 11.3
32 to 33	337	50.2 ± 12.1
34 to 35	857	52.5 ± 11.2
36 to 37	3153	55.6 ± 12.6
38 to 39	10083	57.4 ± 12.6
40 to 41	13841	59.6 ± 12.6
42 to 43	4797	60.3 ± 12.7
44 to 45	1450	60.4 ± 12.7
46 to 47	492	60.5 ± 13.0

Appendix B-4 Umbilical cord length at various gestational ages. (From Naeye RL: Umbilical cord length: Clinical significance. *J Pediatr* 107:278–281, 1985).

UMBILICAL CORD LENGTH

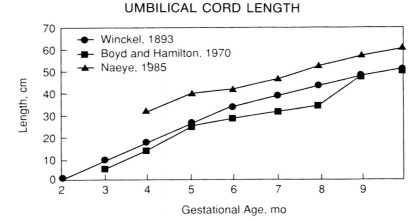

Appendix B-5 Comparison of published cord lengths. (From Benirschke K, Kaufmann P: *Pathology of the Human Placenta.* New York, Springer-Verlag, 1980, p. 194).

REFERENCES

General

Altshuler G: The placenta. In Sternberg SS (ed): *Diagnostic Surgical Pathology.* New York, Raven Press, 1989, p. 1503–1522.

Altshuler G: A conceptual approach to placental pathology and pregnancy outcome. *Sem Diag Pathol* 10:204–221, 1993.

Altshuler G, Hermann AA: The medicolegal imperative: Placenta pathology and epidemiology. In Stevenson DK, Sunshine P (eds): *Fetal and Neonatal Brain Injury: Mechanism, Management, and Risks of Practice.* Philadelphia, B.C. Decker, Inc, 1989, p. 250–263.

Baldwin VJ: Placenta. In Dimmick JE, Kalousek DK (eds): *Developmental Pathology of the Embryo and Fetus.* Philadelphia, JB Lippincott, 1992, p. 271–319.

Benirschke K, Kaufmann P: *Pathology of the Human Placenta.* New York, Springer-Verlag, 1990.

Blanc WA: Pathology of the placenta, membranes and umbilical cord in bacterial, fungal and viral infections in man. In Naeye RL, Kissane JM, Kaufmann N (eds): *Perinatal Diseases.* Baltimore, Williams and Wilkins, 1981, p. 67–132.

Fox H: *Haines and Taylor Obstetrical and Gynaecologic Pathology,* ed 3. New York, Churchill Livingstone, 1987.

Kaplan C, Lowell DM, Salafia C: College of American Pathologists Conference XIX on the examination of the placenta: Report of the working group on the definition of structural changes associated with abnormal function in the maternal/fetal/placental unit in the second and third trimesters. *Arch Pathol Lab Med* 115:709–716, 1991.

Macpherson TA, Szulman AE: The placenta and products of conception. In Silverberg SG (ed): *Principles and Practice of Surgical Pathology,* ed 2. New York, Churchill Livingstone, 1990, 1825–1856.

Naeye RL: *Disorders of the Placenta, Fetus, and Neonate: Diagnosis and Clinical Significance.* St. Louis, Mosby, 1992.

Perrin EVDK: *Pathology of the Placenta.* New York, Churchill Livingstone, 1984.

Examination

Altshuler G, Deppisch LM: College of American Pathologists Conference XIX on the examination of the placenta: Report of the working group on indications for placental examination. *Arch Pathol Lab Med* 115:701–703, 1991.

Clarson C, Tevaarwerk GJM, Harding PGR, et al: Placental weight in diabetic pregnancies. *Placenta* 10:275–281, 1989.

Driscoll SG, Langston C: College of American Pathologists Conference XIX on the examination of the placenta: Report of the working group on methods for placental examination. *Arch Pathol Lab Med* 115:704–708, 1991.

Khong TY, Chambers HM: Alternative method of sampling placentas for the assessment of uteroplacental vasculature. *J Clin Pathol* 45:925–927, 1992.

Manci EA, Ulmer RD, Holland SD et al: Value of clinical, gross, and combined criteria in selection of placentas for microscopic examination. *Mod Pathol* 3:55p, 1990.

Salafia CM, Vintzileos AM: Why all placentas should be examined by a pathologist in 1990. *Am J Obstet Gynecol* 163:1282–1293, 1990.

Development/Vascular Disease

Anderson WR, Davis J: Placental site involution. *Am J Obstet Gynecol* 102:23–33, 1968.

Arias F, Rodriquez L, Rayne SC, et al: Maternal placental vasculopathy and infection: Two distinct subgroups among patients with preterm labor and preterm ruptured membranes. *Am J Obstet Gynecol* 168:585–591, 1993.

Kurman RJ: The morphology, biology, and pathology of intermediate trophoblast: A look back to the present. *Hum Pathol* 22:847–855, 1991.

Naeye RL: Pregnancy hypertension, placental evidences of low uteroplacental blood flow, and spontaneous premature delivery. *Hum Pathol* 20: 441–444, 1989.

Robertson WB, Khong TY, Brosens I, et al: The placental bed biopsy: Review from 3 European centers. *Am J Obstet Gynecol* 155:401–412, 1986.

Umbilical Cord

Clapp JF, Peress NS, Wesley M, et al. Brain damage after intermittent partial cord occlusion in the chronically instrumented fetal lamb. *Am J Obstet Gynecol* 159:504–509, 1988.

Heifetz SA: Single umbilical artery. A statistical analysis of 237 cases and review of the literature. *Perspect Pediatr Pathol* 8:345–378, 1984.

Heifetz SA: Thrombosis of the umbilical cord: Analysis of 52 cases and literature review. *Pediatr Pathol* 8:37–54, 1988.

Hyde S, Smotherman J, Moore JI, et al: A model of bacterially induced umbilical vein spasm, relevant to fetal hypoperfusion. *Obstet Gynecol* 73: 966–970, 1989.

Jacques SM, Qureshi F: Necrotizing funisitis: A study of 45 cases. *Hum Pathol* 23:1278–1283, 1992.

Strong TH, Elliott JP, Radin TG: Non-coiled umbilical blood vessels: A new marker for the fetus at risk. *Obstet Gynecol* 81:409–411, 1993.

Membranes

Altshuler G, Hyde S: Meconium induced vasocontraction: A potential cause of cerebral and other fetal hypoperfusion and of poor pregnancy outcome. *J Child Neurol* 4:137–142, 1989.

Altshuler G, Arizawa M, Molnar-Nadasdy: Meconium induced umbilical cord vascular necrosis and ulceration: A potential link between the placenta and poor pregnancy outcome. *Obstet Gynecol* 79:760–766, 1992.

Gibbs RS, Romero R, Hillier SL, et al: A review of premature birth and subclinical infection. *Am J Obstet Gynecol* 166:1515–1528, 1992.

Miller PW, Coen RW, Benirschke K: Dating the time interval from meconium passage to birth. *Obstet Gynecol* 66:459–462, 1985.

Naeye RL: The clinical significance of absent subchorionic fibrin in the placenta. *Am J Clin Pathol* 94:196–198, 1990.

Naftolin F, Khudr G, Benirschke K, et al: The syndrome of chronic abruptio placentae, hydrorrhea, and circumvallate placenta. *Am J Obstet Gynecol* 116:347–350, 1973.

Romero R, Salafia CM, Athanassiadis AP, et al: The relationship between acute inflammatory lesions of the preterm placental and amniotic fluid microbiology. *Am J Obstet Gynecol* 166:1382–1388, 1992.

Placenta/Villous Lesions

Altshuler G: Chorangiosis: An important placental sign of neonatal morbidity and mortality. *Arch Pathol Lab Med* 108:71–74, 1984.

Andres RL, Kuyper BA, Resnik R, et al: The association of maternal floor infarction of the placenta with adverse perinatal outcome. *Am J Obstet Gynecol* 163:935–938, 1990.

Darby MJ, Caritis SN, Shen-Schwartz S: Placental abruption in the preterm gestation: an association with chorioamnionitis. *Obstet Gynecol* 74:88–92, 1989.

Genest DR, Williams MA, Green MF: Estimating the time of death in stillborn fetuses: II. Histologic evaluation of the placenta: a study of 71 stillborns. *Obstet Gynecol* 80:585–592, 1992.

Gersell DJ: Chronic villitis, chronic chorioamnionitis, and maternal floor infarction. *Sem Diagn Pathol* 10:251–266, 1993.

Kraus FT: Placental thrombi and related problems. *Sem in Diagn Pathol* 10:275–283, 1993.

Machin GA: Hydrops revisited: Literature review of 1414 cases published in the 1980's. *Am J Med Genet* 34:366–390, 1989.

Twins

Baldwin VJ: Pathology of multiple gestation. In Wigglesworth JS, Singer DB (eds): *Textbook of Fetal and Perinatal Pathology.* Boston, Blackwell Scientific, 1990, pp. 221–262.

Baldwin VS: *Pathology of Multiple Pregnancy.* New York. Springer-Verlag, 1993.

Behar R, Vigliocco G, Gramajo H, et al: Antenatal origin of neurologic damage in newborn infants. II. Multiple gestation. *Am J Obstet Gynecol* 162:1230–1236, 1990.

Benirschke K: Intrauterine death of a twin: Mechanisms, implications for surviving twin and placental pathology. *Sem in Diagn Pathol* 10:222–231.

Carr SR, Aronson MP, Coustan DR: Survival rates of monoamniotic twins do not decrease after 30 weeks gestation. *Am J Obstet Gynecol* 163:719–722, 1990.

DeLia JE, Cruikshank DP, Kaye WR: Fetoscopic neodymium:YAG laser occlusion of placental vessels in severe twin-to-twin transfusion syndrome. *Obstet Gynecol* 75:1046–1053, 1990.

Eberle AM, Levesque D, Vintzileos AM, et al. Placental pathology in discordant twins. *Am J Obstet Gynecol* 169:931–935, 1993.

Fusi L, McParland P, Fisk N, et al: Acute twin-twin transfusion: A possible mechanism for brain-damaged survivors after intrauterine death of a monochorionic twin. *Obstet Gynecol* 78:517–520, 1991.

Gavriil P, Jauniaux E, Leroy F: Pathologic examination of placentas from singleton and twin pregnancies obtained after in vitro fertilization and embryo transfer. *Pediatr Pathol* 13:453–462, 1993.

Grafe MR: Antenatal cerebral necrosis in monochorionic twins. *Pediatr Pathol* 13:15–19, 1993.

Scheller JM, Nelson KB: Twinning and neurologic morbidity. *AJDC* 146:1110–1113, 1992.

INDEX